Reflective Practice
for Healthcare
Professionals

Third edition

Reflective Practice for Healthcare Professionals:

A Practical Guide

Third edition

Beverley Joan Taylor

Open University Press

Open University Press
McGraw-Hill Education
McGraw-Hill House
Shoppenhangers Road
Maidenhead
Berkshire
England
SL6 2QL

email: enquiries@openup.co.uk
world wide web: www.openup.co.uk

and Two Penn Plaza, New York, NY 10121-2289, USA

First published 2006
Reprinted 2011

A catalogue record of this book is available from the British Library

ISBN13: 978 0 335 23835 4 (pb)
ISBN10: 0 335 23835 1 (pb)

Library of Congress Cataloging-in-Publication Data
CIP data applied for

Typeset by RefineCatch Limited, Bungay, Suffolk
Printed in the UK by Bell & Bain Ltd, Glasgow

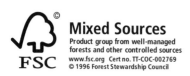

Mixed Sources
Product group from well-managed
forests and other controlled sources
www.fsc.org Cert no. TT-COC-002769
© 1996 Forest Stewardship Council
FSC

The **McGraw·Hill** *Companies*

In loving memory of my mother, Johanna Regina Joan Bugg (née Kennedy) (24 December 1923–6 December 2008), who gave me many opportunities for personal reflection and my love of words and music.

Contents

Introduction

When Open University Press contacted me to invite me to write the third edition of this book, my first impulse was to decline the offer, because I planned to retire from academic work in October 2008, and after almost 40 years of full time labour in the workforce all I could contemplate was taking life a lot easier. My decision to retire was well considered and from my fiftieth birthday, over a five-year period, I began to prepare myself and others for my inevitable disappearance into blissful obscurity.

The 'retiring' phase of my life was a deep source of personal reflection, especially as it was a time of my mother's failing health, while I was trying to have my work responsibilities neatly stored away, with everything completed or handed over. It is true that 'all things come to an end' and my mother died two months after my academic career finished. Mum encouraged me to 'go nursing', she and Dad bought me a little red suitcase to take with me, and Mum wrote me letters from home every week of my three-year training period. I am grateful to them both for getting me started on my nursing career, which led ultimately to academia. I am also grateful for the encouragement and support I received from Open University Press to embark one more time on continuing the tradition of this book, to indulge my abiding love for reflective practice and tie off my academic career neatly.

As an inclusive measure, this book broadens its focus to all healthcare professionals, based on feedback I have received from colleagues in psychology, social work, physiotherapy, medicine, energetic healing and art therapy, about the need for a practical book on reflective practice with wide appeal. As definitions of 'profession' vary, I have taken a baseline approach that a profession has its own knowledge, skills, educational system and codes of conduct and operates with some degree of autonomy. I have left open to the practitioners within the respective fields the final judgement as to the professional status of their developed occupation. The practice stories exemplifying reflective practice have been developed from discussions with various healthcare professionals, who have graciously shared their work experiences with me. Thank you, one and all.

The ability to reflect is evident in human communication and action. With this in mind, this edition guides you through technical, practical and emancipatory reflection using purposeful questioning and openness to possible answers. My personal assumptions in writing this book are that the quality of reflection lies in people's willingness to enquire into their existence in private and public arenas, in order to understand and improve who they are and how they relate to other humans. I am also of the opinion that self-work underlies reflective practice, because to be an effective practitioner at work, one needs to be self-aware and 'at home' in oneself. With this assumption in mind, for the first time, this edition includes my personal reflections on how I am becoming increasingly self-aware, describing some experiences of my life, work and subsequent retirement, to show how becoming more 'at home' with myself in every sphere of my life has complemented my ability to be a reflective person and practitioner. The 'Author's reflections' in this book are accounts of some experiences that have instructed me in living and working, and I offer them to you as examples and possibilities, not as absolutes and prescriptions.

My self-work is essentially based in the ordinariness of being human. I learned most of what it means to be human in my earliest years in my family, where I now realize I first experienced the authenticity of being ordinary, in the sense of interacting with other humans in genuine, commonplace every-dayness. Decades later, when I undertook a PhD, the project illuminated the ordinariness of nurse–patient interactions, and the therapeutic potential of being 'yourself' in healthcare, backed solidly with knowledge, skills and humanity. This edition offers ordinariness as humanness applied broadly to all healthcare professions, as a model of care to augment self-work and human ways of being a reflective practitioner.

The decision to include my PhD research on ordinariness in this edition is inspired by Carmen, who wrote a reflective topical autobiography of her experiences of living with cancer. Her husband Michael and brother Victor accepted the posthumous PhD award on Carmen's behalf in May 2009. In the trajectory of events leading to Carmen's eventual death after seven years in the healthcare system, there was a constant theme of searching for healthcare professionals who could see beyond the problems and treatments of her disease, to Carmen, the intelligent woman with a loving, deeply spiritual core, needing to be informed and involved in her own care. Healthcare professionals were sometimes rough, rude and thoughtless, but for the most part polite and safe. However, the one thing they all had in common was their inability to connect deeply with Carmen. As a model of care, ordinariness does not guarantee increased depths of human connection in every case, but used consciously with the reflective practice processes in this book, I hope that it increases the likelihood that more people receiving healthcare, unlike Carmen, will feel acknowledged, heard and comforted as intelligent human beings.

There are many delights in store for you in this book. Chapter 1 introduces you to the nature of reflection and practice, by describing definitions and perspectives, criticisms, types and sources of reflection. Health professionals are paid to care for people, so this chapter also discusses the nature of caring in health professions, by responding to the questions: What is caring? What is professionalized caring? Why do professionals care? Even though health professionals may espouse caring values, it is not always easy to deliver quality care, so this chapter describes the nature of professional work constraints and suggests that, even against the difficulties, it is still possible to ensure quality practice through reflective processes.

In Chapter 2 I describe some qualities and hints for reflecting, and guide you through your first systematic reflective task, so that you can experience reflective processes first hand. I also describe the role of a critical friend, to help you to reflect at deeper levels, and I explain that this is a role you can adopt in helping others to become more effective in their reflective practice. Finally, I present the 'Taylor model of reflection', using the mnemonic device REFLECT, to give you an easy to remember and apply approach to systematic reflection in your work.

Chapter 3 sounds a note of caution about the use of categories, before introducing three types of reflection you can use in your work, and adapt to your personal life if you wish. Empirical, interpretive and critical knowledge are connected to Habermas' 'knowledge-constitutive interests' to create technical, practical and emancipatory reflection. The relative merits and shortcomings of the types of reflection are described, to assist you in choosing the types to use for your practice. Lastly, I describe a model for being human in healthcare encounters, which can be combined with reflective processes to enhance your knowledge, skills and humanity in your practice.

Chapter 4 reviews information connected directly to technical reflection, including the reasons why this process is used for specific purposes and why it creates different outcomes in terms of knowledge of, and practical answers to, clinical problems. The relationships are explained between empirical knowledge and the scientific method, and how technical reflection fits with these ideas. The connections between technical reflection and evidence-based practice are described and you will find that the two processes are highly complementary. The chapter also describes the technical reflection process, practice stories, critical friend responses and other examples of how technical reflection can be used by reflective healthcare professionals.

In Chapter 5 I review some information connected directly to practical reflection, and in Chapter 6 I review some information connected directly to emancipatory reflection, before guiding you through the respective reflection process, practice stories, critical friend responses and other examples of how the type of reflection can be used by healthcare professionals.

Chapter 7 encourages you to apply the REFLECT model to your own healthcare practice, so that you can become accustomed to reflecting on your own practice stories, in order to make sense of them and make any necessary changes. Bearing in mind the busyness of healthcare professionals, I present the model in an abbreviated, point-form guide, which you can use easily and comprehensively in your workplace or at home.

Chapter 8 provides practical information on how to incorporate reflective practice into research methodologies and scholarship in the form of healthcare knowledge. Reflective methods and processes fit well with all qualitative research methodologies, and this chapter identifies possible applications before focusing on specific projects involving action research. The chapter also describes how to foster scholarship by preparing your research findings for conference presentations and journal articles, because research worth doing is worth sharing to improve practice and to extend interdisciplinary knowledge.

In the final chapter, I reiterate the importance being human in your profession, while maintaining the high standards of knowledge and skills required to practise safely and authentically. I suggest some ways of maintaining reflective practice by affirming yourself as a reflective practitioner, responding to the critiques, creating a daily habit, seeing things freshly, staying alert to practice, finding support systems, sharing reflection, getting involved in research and embodying reflective practice.

So, welcome to this book and to reflection in your personal and professional life. My sincere hope is you will never be quite the same again after reading this book.

BJ Taylor

1 The nature of reflection and practice

Introduction

As far as we can ascertain, humans are the only beings on earth with the ability to engage in deep internal thought processes and to activate those thoughts outwardly in language and action. Humans have the potential to think, and to think about thinking, because our higher order cognition involves memory and reflection. In this sense, cognition sets us above all other species of animals and it is the means by which we direct our intentions outwards, towards other humans, animals, plants and the physical world of matter. We can also turn our thoughts inwards towards the intrapersonal self, making sense of moment-to-moment events, our lives and our relationships with other people, and the contexts in which we interact. Our inner world of thoughts governs who we are and who we are becoming – for example, by perpetuating self-limiting thoughts, or by engaging in opening ourselves up to imagining unlimited possibilities. We can contemplate abstractions, such as infinity and the possibility of worlds beyond worlds, through our ability to imagine and reflect on ideas.

Thinking can be employed in our daily lives to maintain our beliefs, values, routines, rituals and habits and to orientate us towards our personal goals. For example, we can choose to stay the way we are, or to work consciously towards changing ourselves. Thinking gives us some degree of control over our own moods and attitudes, if we are willing to reflect on how emotions and beliefs affect us and other people around us. For example, we can choose to convert a 'bad mood' into a 'good mood', or use our internal dialogues to determine if we are 'a glass half full' or a 'glass half empty' type of person.

This book emphasizes your thinking in the workplace, as a reflective health professional. Even though the focus is on your work as a professional within healthcare settings, the book also engages you in reflection on yourself as a human being. To these ends, this chapter introduces you to the nature of reflection and practice, by describing definitions and perspectives, criticisms, types and sources of reflection. Health professionals are paid to care for people, so this chapter also discusses the nature of caring in health professions by responding to the questions: What is caring? What is professionalized caring? Why do professionals care? Even though health professionals may espouse caring values, it is not always easy to deliver quality care, so this chapter describes the nature of professional work constraints and suggests that, even against the difficulties, it is still possible to ensure quality practice through reflective processes.

Definitions and perspectives of reflection

In the physical world, reflection means throwing back from a surface, such as that creating heat, sound or light. In connection with human reflection, I extend the definition to the throwing back of thoughts and memories, in cognitive acts such as thinking, contemplation, meditation and any other form of attentive consideration, in order to make sense of them, and to make contextually appropriate changes if they are required (Taylor 2000: 3). This comprehensive definition allows for a wide variety of thinking as the basis for reflection, but it is similar to many other explanations (Mezirow 1981; Boyd and Fales 1983; Boud *et al.* 1985; Street 1992) due to the inclusion of the two main aspects of thinking as a rational and intuitive process, which allows the potential for change.

The most notable name in the educational reflective practice literature is Donald Schön, who emphasized the idea that reflection is a way in which professionals can bridge the theory–practice gap, based on the potential of reflection to uncover knowledge in and on action (Schön 1983). He acknowledged the working intelligence of practitioners, and their potential to make sense of their work in a theoretical way, even though they might tend to underestimate their practical knowledge. He referred to 'tacit knowledge', or 'knowing in action', as the kind of knowledge of which they may not be entirely aware. Tacit knowledge becomes embodied and effortless to practitioners, so they become relatively unaware of their implicit expertise.

When practitioners, such as healthcare professionals, are coached to make their knowing in action explicit, they can inevitably use this awareness to enliven and change their practice (Schön 1987). Interestingly, this assumes that reflection is not a natural state, known without introduction, to all people who engage in practice. Schön realized that systematic processes need to be guided experiences, so that practitioners can derive the best possible outcomes from them. This means that healthcare professionals need assistance in identifying and describing their workplace practices, in order to maximize what they do well and remedy those behaviours in need of amendment and change. Thus, reflection addresses the fundamental issues in effective healthcare.

Reflector

Is your practice effective in every respect? What do you do well? What could you do better?

Argyris and Schön (1974) and Argyris *et al.* (1985) suggested that practitioners often practise at less than effective levels, because they follow routine. Furthermore, their actual practice does not necessarily coincide with their 'better knowledge' or espoused theories about good practice. In fact, as Kim (1999) suggests, they may not even be aware of this divergence. Praxis is different practice as a result of reflection, which encompasses a change in the status quo (Taylor 2000). As Kim (1999: 4) states:

> practitioners can engage in self-dialogue and argumentation with themselves in order to clarify validity claims embedded in their actions, bringing forth the hidden meanings and disguises that systematically result in self-oriented and unilateral actions or ineffective habitual forms of practice.

This means that healthcare professionals can use reflective processes to identify the 'truth' of what they do, so they can recognize the traps they fall into routinely, in resorting to unexamined habits to get them through their work. This form of reflection allows you to firstly identify the habit, then see it in a different light, by interrogating the purposes it serves and why you continue to perpetuate the habit, so that you can begin to change your practices. You may now see why Schön (1987) was of the opinion that reflection is not a natural state and why practitioners need help to guide them in reflecting systematically.

Previously, the practice disciplines of nursing and midwifery have applied reflective practice ideas to many of their work areas (Taylor 2000, 2006). For example, in nursing, reflective practice has been used successfully in practice and practice development (Taylor 2000, 2002a, 2002b; Thorpe and Barsky 2001; Stickley and Freshwater 2002; Johns 2003), clinical supervision (Todd and Freshwater 1999; Heath and Freshwater 2000; Gilbert 2001), and education (Cruickshank 1996; Freshwater 1999a, 1999b; Kim 1999; Anderson and Branch 2000; Clegg 2000; Platzer *et al.* 2000a, 2000b). These areas have been described fully in these and other important publications (Bolton 2005; Ghaye and Lillyman 2006; Freshwater *et al.* 2008).

Increasingly, reflective practice is being applied to diverse fields of human endeavour, such as architecture (Dimendberg and Lerup 2002) engineering (Dyck 1997), politics (Goodin 2005; United Nations Centre for Human Settlements 2005; Normore 2009), organizations and institutions (Day *et al.* 2001; Wilson 2005; Morgan 2006; Senge 2006; Rustin and Bradley 2008), business, management and leadership (Burgoyne and Reynolds 1997; Golding and Currie 2000; Chaharbaghi 2004; Beirne 2006; Brown 2006; Segal 2006; Cartwright 2007; Pellicer 2007; Griffin 2008) and environment and sustainability issues (Clarke and Reading 1994; Thomashow 1996; Azapagic *et al.* 2004; Wessels 2006).

Reflective practice also continues to grow in areas devoted to human helping, such as health and human services (Sternberg and Horvath 1999; Drinka and Clark 2000; Gardner and Boucher 2000; Murray and Simpson 2000; Young and Cooke 2002; Jasper 2003; McDermott 2003; Bolton 2005; Ghaye 2005; Bradley 2006; Ghaye and Lillyman 2006; Redmond 2006; Webb 2006; Cherry 2008; McKinlay and Ross 2008) and religious roles and practices (Munson 1976; Carroll 1986; Carroll and Carroll 1991; Fitzgerald 1993; Sik 1997; Gelpi 1998; Chadwick and Tovey 2001; Hughes 2001; Kitchen 2002; Miller 2007; Oliver 2007).

In healthcare professions other than nursing and midwifery, where it has been in use for some time, reflective practice has been adopted by psychology and counselling (Shapiro 1985; Hoshmand 1994; Osofsky and Fitzgerald 1999; Hughes 2001; Beres 2002; Mickelson 2002; Swartz *et al.* 2002; Ekman 2004; Hoare 2006; Renninger and Sigel 2006; Harms 2007; Corey 2008), social work (Yelloly and Henkel 1995; Gould and Taylor 1996; Martyn and Atkinson 2000; Poulter 2001; Davies 2002; Cooper *et al.* 2003; Gould and Baldwin 2004; Robb *et al.* 2004; Ruch 2004; Dolan *et al.* 2006; Knott and Scragg 2007; Warren-Adamson and Ruch 2008; Hookins *et al.* 2009), occupational therapy (Kinsella 2000; Couch 2004) and medicine (Daniels 1996; MacAuley, *et al.* 1998; Leyden 2004; Doyle *et al.* 2005; Soares 2005; Pitts 2007) .

Reflection in psychology includes phenomenological psychology of human existence and bodily sense (Shapiro 1985), orientation to inquiry in reflective professional psychology (Hoshmand 1994), reflective practice with abused women (Beres 2002), the social construction of reflective practice (Mickelson 2002), psychodynamic ideas in the South African community (Swartz *et al.* 2002), recognizing faces and feelings to improve communication and emotional life (Ekman 2004), and multidimensional approaches to understanding the complexities of an individual's experience, to help experienced practitioners to think critically and to reflect on practice (Harms 2007).

Reflection in relation to human development includes Osofsky and Fitzgerald's (1999) *Handbook of Infant Mental Health* and Hughes's (2001) exploration of the complexities of children's play, emphasizing the necessity of adult-free play for the psychological well-being of the child. Hoare (2006) includes reflective practice in a handbook, which brings together the leading scholars from adult development and learning to explore six major aspects of foundations, key areas of integration, the self system, higher reaches of development and learning, essential contexts and specific applications. Renninger and Sigel (2006) include reflection when they span the entire field of child development, including spirituality, social understanding and non-verbal communication. In counselling, Corey (2008) encourages counsellors to use reflection to develop their own style, and Dallos and Stedmon (2009) describe *Reflective Practice in Psychotherapy and Counselling*.

Considerable advances have been made in incorporating reflective practice into social work, for example, in learning and teaching in social work (Yelloly and Henkel 1995; Gould and Taylor 1996; Martin and Atkinson 2000; Davies 2002; Gould and Baldwin 2004) and modern social work theory (Payne and Campling 2005) including reflection inherent in anti-oppressive practice, ecological systems theory and postmodern feminism. Reflection also features in social work issues involving children (Poulter 2001; Cooper *et al.* 2003; Ruch 2004; Warren-Adamson and Ruch 2008) and family support (Dolan *et al.* 2006).

Robb *et al.* (2004) describe communication and relationships, which have become an increasing focus of attention in debates about the future of health and social care. They encourage people working in healthcare to improve communication processes, to develop more participatory relationships with service users and to work more closely in partnership with other professionals. Knott and Scragg (2007) describe reflective practice as a key learning and development process, including emotionally intelligent workers, dangerousness, men in social work, interprofessional leadership and maintaining and enhancing reflection in the workplace, and Hookins *et al.* (2009) also provide guidance in *Developing Reflective Practice in Social Work: A Critical Approach*.

Key publications in reflective practice in occupational therapy include *Professional Development and Reflective Practice* (Kinsella 2000) and *Reflective Practice in Occupational Therapy* (Couch 2004).

In medicine, publications making mention of reflection include the *Oxford Textbook of Palliative Medicine* (Doyle *et al.* 2005) and a wide-ranging collection of essays by a medical ethicist in the USA exploring the claim that justification in ethics in theory or practice involves achieving coherence or 'reflective equilibrium' (Daniels 1996). More specifically, MacAuley *et al.* (1998) provide a guide to reflective practice for qualifying GPs and other healthcare professionals, Pitts (2007) describes *Portfolios, Personal Development and Reflective Practice*, Leyden (2004) targets *Primary Care Physicians in Reflective Practice: Learning to Treat Depression* and Soares (2005) informs practitioners on *Reflective Practice in Medicine*.

Reflector

Who are the key authors in reflective practice in your healthcare profession? You can check by opening Google Scholar and/or Google Books on your internet service. Enter the keywords 'reflective practice' and the title of your profession. On what areas are these publications focusing? To what extent do these publications teach you about how to be a reflective practitioner in your work?

This section has introduced you to various definitions and perspectives of reflection. From its beginnings in education with the work of Donald Schön, reflective practice has been taken up by many fields of human endeavour, such as engineering, environment and sustainability, politics, organizations and architecture. In human health and helping services the literature shows that mainly nursing, midwifery, psychology and counselling, social work, occupational therapy and medicine have embraced reflective practice. All of these human agencies agree that reflective practice improves work satisfaction, processes and outcomes. Thoughtfulness and purposeful communication and action reside at the heart of what matters in effective practice. This being so, this book provides another important source of practical guidance in knowing yourself better and improving your practices in your healthcare profession.

Criticisms of reflective practice

Even though it has proved successful, critics have perceived limitations in reflective practice. For example, in nursing, where reflective practice has long since moved past its 'honeymoon phase', critics have pointed out how the profession seized on the idea of reflection (Jarvis 1992), that a high degree of personal investment is required for successful practice outcomes (Taylor 1997), barriers to learning must be overcome before midwives and nurses reflect effectively (Platzer *et al.* 2000b), there may be cultural barriers to empowerment through reflection (Johns 1999), negative consequences may ensue when practitioners are pressured to reflect (Hulatt 1995), reflection is a fundamentally flawed strategy (Mackintosh 1998), there are potential dangers in promoting 'private thoughts in public spheres' (Cotton 2001), reflective processes have failed to 'address the postmodern, cultural contexts of reflection' (Pryce 2002), and there is a lack of research evidence to support the mandate to reflect (Burton 2000).

Ghaye and Lillyman (2000) critically reviewed the foundations and criticisms of reflective practice to question whether reflective practitioners were really 'fashion victims', and having explored the limitations of it, concluded that reflective practice has a place in the postmodern world, because of its ability to explore micro levels of human interaction and personal knowledge. Contrastingly, Taylor (2003: 244) argued that 'reflective practice tends to adopt a naïve or romantic realist position and fails to acknowledge the ways in which reflective accounts construct the world of practice'.

Reflector

List some examples of 'micro levels of human interaction and personal knowledge' in your healthcare profession. What are the advantages and disadvantages in exploring these micro levels?

Nurses have responded directly to critics (e.g. Sargent 2001; Markham 2002; Rolfe 2003) and in spite of the concerns and critiques, clinicians, educators and researchers tend to agree that although reflective practice has its limitations, and requires time, effort and ongoing commitment, it is nevertheless worth the effort to bring about deeper insights and changes in practice, leadership, clinical supervision and education.

Reflector

Is there any criticism of reflective practice in your healthcare profession's literature? On an anecdotal level, how do professionals in your healthcare discipline talk about reflective practice? If there is resistance to reflective practice, what are the main arguments?

Types of reflection

Once committed to a life of reflection, it takes time and effort to maintain a reflective approach. In this book I reiterate my position that it simplifies the enormous task of thinking about reflection if we imagine that there are three main types of reflection useful for people engaged in any kind of practice: technical, practical and emancipatory reflection.

Technical reflection, based on the scientific method and rational, deductive thinking, will allow you to generate and validate empirical knowledge through rigorous means, so that you can be assured that work procedures are based on scientific reasoning. This means that you will develop an objective method for working out how to make policies and procedures better, by exposing your technical work issues to systematic questioning and coherent argumentation and revision. For example, you may want to update a procedure, or argue whether a policy is still appropriate. Technical reflection gives you the knowledge and skills of critical thinking and provides a framework for questioning, which results in an objective, well-argued position to support any adaptations and improvements needed.

Practical reflection leads to interpretation for description and explanation of human interaction in social existence. This simply means that you can use this type of reflection to improve the way you communicate with other people at work, thereby improving your practice enjoyment and outcomes. For example, you may identify a dysfunctional communication pattern with other staff, such as peers and allied staff. Practical reflection provides a systematic questioning process that encourages you to reflect deeply on role relationships, to locate their dynamics and habitual issues, so that changes can be made to improve communication.

Emancipatory reflection leads to 'transformative action', which seeks to free you from taken-for-granted assumptions and oppressive forces, which limit you and your practice. In other words, this type of reflection lets you see what subtle and not so subtle powerful forces and circumstances are holding you back from achieving your goals. When you have an increased awareness, you have taken the first step in making some changes in the ways you think about and overcome these constraints. For example, you may identify powerlessness at work in relation to making clinical decisions. Emancipatory reflection provides a systematic questioning process to help you to locate the bases of the problem, identify the constraints and begin to address the issues, either alone or through collaborative action with other healthcare professionals.

Work and life issues and challenges do not fit easily into regular, fixed compartments, so I make the point now, and reiterate later, that the types of reflection can be used alone or in any combination you choose, to address the work issues in your practice. All kinds of knowledge can be generated through reflection and healthcare professionals can benefit from a range of reflective processes.

Sources of reflection

Life is a source of reflection, because it is an energized process through which humans are embodied to live daily as individuals and act in relation to other people and contexts. Taking an active interest in life through reflection turns one's existence into something more than the mere passing of time. When life and all of its expressions, such as events, circumstances, symbols and relationships with other people and our environments come into clearer and finer focus, life has the potential to be more meaningful. Plato was so convinced of the power of reflection that he declared 'The unreflected life is not worth living'. While death seems a severe alternative to thoughtlessness, reflection can turn an unconsidered life into an existence, which is consciously aware, self-potentiating and purposeful.

Within human existence, traditions and rituals become sustained over time, such as work and leisure, philosophies, disciplines, art and religious beliefs. These form rich sources of reflection and they can in turn facilitate further reflection. Unpaid and paid work hours may take up significant time in the overall time apportioned to a human life, so if reflective attention is focused on work rituals, habits and routines, the drudgery and obligation to pay the bills or fill in idle time can be transformed into life and work insights and changes. Leisure time can be given over to thoughtfulness, as time and space is taken to reflect outside the recurrent demands of work responsibilities, because you are always 'a work in progress'.

Philosophies share the love of knowledge and philosophers ask the perennial question: What is existence and what is knowledge? This question and associated enquiries is asked over and over in new circles, in the light of previously reflected and debated positions, to create new paradigms. Through reflection, disciplines such as philosophy and sociology continually generate ever-increasing and refined knowledge. Practice disciplines, such as healthcare professions, use reflection to identify and refine their practice bases and to find meaning in the work.

Through the inspiration of creativity and reflection, artists of all kinds create novel representations of life, such as paintings, pottery, ceramics, music, sculpture, literature and poetry. Art comes from a creative and thoughtful source and we respond to it through a similar process, as it 'speaks' to us. Novel images, textures, sounds and forms are assimilated into the repertoire of 'givens' in our lives in that very moment we experience them through our senses, making the unfamiliar familiar through an instantaneous reflective awareness. Just as we find every human face familiar as we take our first fleeting glimpse, so we have the capacity to 'take on board' newness, strangeness and difference in the flash of a thought.

Through religious and spiritual practices, humans reflect on the nature of human life and its potential connections with higher consciousness. World religions of all faiths and denominations differ in their definitions of a supreme entity, although they agree that a sense of daily closeness to that entity comes through some form of reflection and supplication. Because humans have the capacity for thought, they also have the potential to imagine something or someone greater than themselves.

Reflector

What are the sources of reflection in your life? It may help to jot down a few ideas and think about why these sources of reflection have been helpful to you.

There is value in reflection, which comes from the process of thinking itself and the possibilities that engagement offers. Imagine a world in which all actions towards people and the environment are unconsidered and the outcomes of those actions are unreflected. What happens to social order and welfare in an unreflected human existence? Even when people have strong moral bases and nations appear to have well-developed social consciences, inequalities, prejudice, greed, famine, genocide, wars and other crimes against humanity still occur. At this worldwide level, reflection becomes the basis for history, the present, and the future. If people do not consider the events of their past, they are unable to take advantage of the present and powerless to shape their future, because they will remain oblivious to patterns, habits, trends and forces that shape their lives and those of the wider human community.

In this book I place a strongly positive light on the value of reflection, because it has the potential for making sense of the past and present, to project you forward into a more considered future as a person and as a worker. Healthcare professionals are busy people, who work hard in their daily work. I am of the opinion that if you become convinced of the value of reflection in your life and work, and that if you take time to practise reflective thinking as an everyday habit, you will experience personal and professional benefits. Reflection is not magical; it is a daily commitment to thinking systematically and purposefully, to raise your awareness and potentiate positive changes.

Author's reflection

In the introduction to this book, I explained that this edition is inclusive of all healthcare professions and that I am of the opinion that self-work is fundamental to reflective practice. Wishing to exemplify the connections between self-work and reflective practice, this is the first in a series of my reflections throughout this book, sharing with you my thoughts about how I have developed reflection in my personal life and permeated my reflective identity into my clinical and academic work.

Looking back to my early life memories, I can see now that I was always a thoughtful kind of child. This did not necessarily make me a 'good child', because I had my fair share of naughtiness and, together with my brothers and sister, I provided my parents with plenty of challenges. However, below the microanalyses of daily events and minor calamities, I had a calm, unshakeable sense of my deep, internal self.

One of my retirement projects now is to write my autobiography, entitled *Snow on Cradle*. 'It's so cold today, there must be snow on Cradle'; that is what my father would say when we were greeted by ice sheets on puddles and frost in the air, when I was a child. I grew up in a working-class suburb in Burnie, Tasmania, in the 1950s. I did not recognize it then, that my father's predictions about the weather were to be a metaphor for my life. My favourite place on earth is Cradle Mountain, overlooking Dove Lake, in north-western Tasmania. If you imagine Tasmania as an inverted triangle, Cradle Mountain and Dove Lake lie like a heart, displaced a little towards the anatomical right side of Tassie's chest.

To give you a sense of who I am, this is an excerpt from the working draft of my autobiography:

> Going back to my earliest memories, I rely on a Box Brownie camera to help me recollect standing in front of a sunny wall. I can feel my

pants pulled right up under my nipples, having no waist landmark to hold them down. My chest is flat, clean and perfect. The air in my lungs is only a few years old, tiny remnants remaining from when I first drew breath on Sunday, the ninth day of September, 1951. I have a sense of feeling loved and protected and I notice that anything I do is received with fondness. I am the most pure I can remember being. I have no guile, no distortions, and no emotions covering layers of emotion. I am me, and it is to this little child I must return often, to remember who I am.

In another photo we kids, Ken, Bobby, Di and I, are out the back yard of our Round Hill home dressed in our Sunday best clothes. I remember the feel of the little tartan skirt and pullover, and the slight pinch of my clean white socks and leather sandals. I am sitting in a cardboard box, with my feet dangling over the side. Di is just to my side, looking cheekily from her vantage point on her three-wheeler trike. Kenny, the eldest, is in the background looking extremely neat and tidy and Bobby, the second eldest, is leaning forward to make sure his wide grin fits into the picture.

Another black and white photo, which conjures memories, is of we four kids at a fancy dress night. Kenny is a Christmas tree. He is wearing a conical green sheath over his entire body with ornaments and streamers pinned to the fabric. He can see where he is going through peepholes at the apex of his outfit. Di is the bride. She has a tired, slightly forlorn look on her face, but she has all the grace and innocence of the Holy Mother, with a white cloth veil following the shape of her head and neck and a little white dress, which she has managed to keep pristine. Bobby is the groom, standing beside Di. He is wearing a little black suit and hat, with wide-eyed apprehension. I was told that Bobby took his role as groom so seriously, that he messed his pants and needed to be taken home for some 'running repairs'. I am the flower girl. The frilled bodice of my white dress barrels my little chest slightly upwards. I have flowers in my silvery hair and my new white socks are turned down neatly just above my ankles. My sandals have been painted silver and the combined effect of the new socks and silver shoes make me think that I can dance on air. I am carrying a silver frosted basket containing fresh flowers and I am trying hard to keep it held in front of me, where every-one can see it, so they know I'm the flower girl. I sense that people think I am lovely. They are looking at me tenderly, making soft, cooing sounds.

At first glance, these touching images of myself may seem sweet, but inconsequential. Over time I have come to see that these memories form the basis of my self-identity and they have a great bearing on how I am discovering who I am and how I have developed personally and professionally. I have been a flower girl in many professional roles throughout my life. Some people have adored my work in nursing and midwifery practice and others have told me how much they have enjoyed reading and applying my academic writing. While accepting their adoration and praise, I have been conscious of keeping my ego in check, finding a balance in notoriety and obscurity, and arrogance and humility. I have nurtured my pure self, tucked away warmly and safely, keeping my childlike sense of awe and wonderment deep inside myself, as a basis for developing my own kind of authenticity in human interactions.

I place a strongly positive light on the value of personal reflection, because it helps me to make sense of my past and present, to project me forward into a more considered future as a person. While I breathe, I learn. I take the time to practise reflective thinking every day, through meditation, gardening and interacting with friends and family, Winnie, our geriatric dog, and Tundra and Chimera, our two cats. As a consequence, I experience the benefits of a deeper sense of self and increasing integration in my academic writing.

The nature of caring in health professions

The complexity of work within the healthcare professions means that it is not a simple job to be effective in your work. With so many tasks, roles, relationships, expectations and unforeseen aspects to negotiate, it is no wonder that practice has a tendency to become chaotic and unpredictable. In the relative madness that makes up a 'good' work day, the least you might hope for is that your work will be safe and polite, and at the very best that it will be therapeutic and genuine. This book envisages helping you move towards therapeutic and genuine practice, by helping you to identify and act on those factors that prevent you from being as effective as you might ideally hope to be on a regular basis at work.

What is caring?

Caring is a well described concept, especially in caring professions, such as nursing and midwifery. Caring has been described as a virtue, a set of human characteristics, and as an undervalued feminine approach. Caring has been applied to disciplines such as medicine, nursing and education, and as a general concept in the division of domestic labour. These areas are explored in this section to build a broad appreciation of the concept and to find applications for reflective healthcare practice.

People tend to use the words 'care' (a noun) and 'caring' (a verb) without reference to their meaning in terms of their intentions and outcomes. For example, as a noun, 'care' is something given or received, such as in medical or nursing care. Regardless of whether care is perceived by either party in the exchange as being good, bad or indifferent, the intention is to impart care and in the process make some sort of difference to the person concerned. As a verb, 'caring' can convey two main intentions, which are 'caring for' and 'caring about' an object of attention, which may be human or non-human. This raises a qualitative difference in, for example, the ways in which you may care for a client and your car. Therefore, you need to be aware of the different uses of the words 'care' and 'caring' and keep them in mind as we progress in this section.

Reflector

In his chapter, 'Caring: an essay in the philosophy of caring', van Hooft explores the word 'care' in the grammatical sense and in relation to literature (van Hooft *et al.* 1995: 29–47). He makes the claim that 'when one acts caringly, one implicates oneself in what one does, and that is what matters' (p. 47). To what extent do you agree or disagree with the statement? How important is authenticity in caring? In other words, is inauthentic caring a contradiction in terms? If so, how is it so?

Caring has been described in terms of the attributes of the caring relationship (Mayeroff 1971), such as knowing, alternating rhythms, patience, honesty, trust, humility, hope and courage. In relation to the characteristics of the carer, Noddings (1984) forwarded the view that caring is a feminine trait derived from feminine emotionality, which results in warm, relational aspects of caring. Care has also been described from an existential perspective as a human standpoint or 'mode of being' from which caring originates and moves towards others (Heidegger 1962).

Probably the most common approach to caring philosophy has been through virtue ethics, which has been differentiated as a desire or inclination to do good, an action which demonstrates goodwill, and the ability to meet prescribed standards (Brody 1988). There are some difficulties with this position. For example, if caring is moral virtue, and a person has a desire to do good and acts with goodwill, can it then be assumed that the resulting action is morally good, regardless of its consequences? Curzer (1993: 51) takes the view 'that care is a vice rather than a virtue' for healthcare professionals and that they 'should not care for their patients' but they 'should be benevolent and act in a caring manner' towards them.

Reflector

Reflect on the advantages and disadvantages of emotional attachment in caring. What degree of closeness do you adopt in caring for others? Why?

Debates have persisted within virtue ethics as to whether caring is a virtue and if so, in what ways. For example, Carol Gilligan (1977, 1982) argued that virtue is located in the action, and she regarded caring as manifested in the 'caring act'. MacIntyre (1984), a philosopher, put the view that virtue is the ability to meet prescribed standards and for healthcare professionals this fits well with the competency standards expected in a caring role. In applying the debate to a theory of nursing ethics, Fry (1989) suggested that caring could not be regarded as a primary virtue in itself, because some kinds of caring are not intrinsically moral, for example, the 'natural caring' between a mother and her child. Interestingly, this view could reduce human caring to a biological instinct with no moral content.

Feminist writers have criticized contemporary society and healthcare systems in which caring is devalued as a feminine trait. Based on the work of Carol Gilligan, a feminist perspective on caring was forwarded by Puka (1990, 1991), who claimed that care has developed as a coping strategy to deal with sexist socialization experiences and that a new model of 'caring as liberation' is required. Noddings (1984) regarded caring as the moral foundation of interpersonal relationships and although this applies equally to men and women, caring is gender relevant and arises from a longing for goodness. For Noddings, caring is not about moral reasoning or theories, but rather 'the ethic of caring' is a value, which involves receptivity, relatedness and responsiveness, all of which result in joy. Critiques of Noddings' work (e.g. Card 1990; Houston 1990; Hoagland 1991) have been along the lines that Noddings' work does not account for the care of strangers, nor the possibility of evil, and that it leaves itself open for exploitation.

Medical practitioners have traditionally focused on the technicalities of care, basing their procedures on empirical research and placing importance on the 'what' of care. Increasingly, discussions of caring not only include the 'what' but also the 'how' of attending to people's healthcare needs. For example, in a call for articles about caring for critically ill patients to be submitted to *The Journal of the American Medical Association*, Cook (1998: 181) wrote the following comments:

> Undeniably, the knowledge, skills, compassion, and resources needed to care for acutely and seriously ill patients transcend more than 2 specialities. Accordingly, we are renaming this section 'Caring for the Ill Patient', in the spirit of the multidisciplinary, holistic perspective championed by numerous disciplines and in venues not limited to emergency departments and intensive care units. The care of critically ill patients will continue to evolve in the next millennium, and contents of this section will mirror this evolution and progress.

Care has been applied as a general concept in many ways. For example, attention has been paid to men as carers in families. A multicultural perspective of men as carers reveals different expectations of how they will care within a family context. In an article about the sexual division of care in mainland China and Hong Kong, Yu and Chau (1997: 607) reported that:

> women in China and Hong Kong are expected to take up more caring responsibilities than men . . . This is similar to women in traditional Chinese society. An important reason is that the political and economic conditions in Hong Kong and mainland China favour the reproduction of traditional Chinese values. Hence it can be argued that the unequal division of domestic labour will continue as long as the political and economic conditions are unfavourable to women.

In contrast, research relating to caring fathers in the Netherlands (Duindam and Spruijt 1997: 149) shows that 'caring men do not report a lesser degree of well-being, including the quality of their relationship'.

Reflector

Caring is central and fundamental to any discussions about healthcare. Locate definitions and descriptions of caring which apply to your healthcare profession. You may be able to locate them rapidly, by opening Google Scholar and using the keywords health/care/(your healthcare profession). How do these authors provide descriptions of caring which are helpful for understanding the kind of work and the nature of interpersonal interactions common to your healthcare profession?

What is professionalized caring?

Caring for the sick varies according to where it is done and by whom. Family members may care for sick relatives in the home for little or no remuneration, whereas healthcare professionals are paid to care for strangers. When caring is based on payment and prestige in return for specialized knowledge and skills it becomes professional.

Healthcare workers identify themselves as professionals, having evolved in their practice from occupational to professional status. Occupations become professions by attaining the credentials of professionalism. The ways in which an occupation transforms itself into a profession vary, but are generally considered to entail a strong level of commitment; a long and disciplined educational process; a unique body of knowledge and skill; discretionary authority and judgement; active and cohesive professional organization; and acknowledged social worth and contribution.

Goode (1966, in Freidson 1970) describes professions according to two core characteristics: 'a prolonged specialized training in a body of abstract knowledge' and 'a collectivity or service orientation', with autonomy for professional standards and education, licensing, legislation and freedom from lay evaluation and control. Freidson, however, argues that the only truly important and uniform criterion for distinguishing professions from other occupations is 'the fact of autonomy – a position of legitimate control over work' (1970: 82). He adds that professionalization often requires the support of powerful groups within the social structure.

Reflector

On what grounds does your healthcare group argue that it has evolved from an occupation to a profession?

Why do professionals care?

Professionalized caring involves working according to specialized knowledge and skills and codes of conduct, to provide healthcare to clients, who pay for the service. Professionals choose to care and they pursue this decision through years of specialized training and education, to develop the skills and knowledge which characterize their chosen field. In return for their efforts, they receive public acknowledgement through suitable remuneration, status and prestige. Intrinsic benefits may follow, for example, in giving the professional a deeper sense of self and life purpose. This kind of professional caring results in earning a living while enjoying the privilege of providing a service to humanity.

Reflector

As we have seen previously, care can be construed as 'care' (a noun) and 'caring' (a verb). For example, as a noun, 'care' is something given or received, such as in medical or nursing care. As a verb, 'caring' can convey 'caring for' and 'caring about' an object of attention. With these distinctions in mind, reflect on the follow questions: What does professional caring mean to you? For whom do you care? Do you care about the people you serve in your healthcare profession?

Summary

Contemporary concepts of caring vary, but they rest mainly on the interpretation of the words 'care' and 'caring' in virtue ethics and by writers from diverse backgrounds, such as philosophy, feminism, education and nursing. Critiques of caring have shown that it is not a simple matter of orientating good intentions towards another person, but that the whole area of caring requires deeper and more sustained enquiry into intentions, processes and outcomes. Care has been applied as a general concept in many ways, for example, in the practice of education, the division of domestic labour in cross-cultural settings, and in relation to men as carers in families. Cultural perspectives of gender responsibilities, and political, economic and historical factors are involved in discussions of care and caring. Reflective healthcare professionals need to be aware of the literature and debates in caring, in order to apply these implications to their practice.

Even though healthcare workers identify themselves as professionals, having attained the credentials of professionalism involving a strong level of commitment, a long and disciplined educational process, a unique body of knowledge and skill, discretionary authority and judgement, active and cohesive professional organization and acknowledged social worth and contribution, they may not necessarily think beyond the obvious features of their work roles and responsibilities.

Systematic approaches to reflection and action are needed to make sense of your personal and professional identity, to enhance the likelihood that your professionalized caring will be effective, given the complexity of your professional knowledge and skills and the nature of daily work constraints.

The nature of work constraints

When you go to work for an employer or engage in private practice you usually step into a context outside the relative comfort and predictability of your own home to interact with other human beings. Work contexts are complex situations where you experience the intersection of different people, and their motives, agendas, and ways of working and interacting, so that routine and unexpected events result in a seemingly endless array of cascading outcomes. With so much happening and with so much at stake in terms of people's health and well-being, it is no wonder that 'things go wrong' in healthcare professions.

After years of working with nurses and midwives I realize that they find it relatively easy to blame themselves when 'things go wrong' at work. There are many reasons why healthcare professionals are 'hard on themselves' and we will go into some of these later. The realization for any healthcare professional that you are not the only reason that things can go wrong in your practice may free you from bitter self-recriminations and raise your awareness to be able to transform some or all of the conditions that constrain you. If you recognize your tendency to blame yourself when things go wrong at work, you may be relieved to know that a careful appraisal of the possible constraints on your work practices can show you that many variables interact to construct a complex situation, and that they can be acknowledged and worked on intentionally and systematically, to improve your work satisfaction and effectiveness. It may help you to think of work constraints as being cultural, economic, historical, political, social and personal, and to understand that they may affect the ways in which you are able to interpret and act at any given moment at work.

Cultural constraints

Cultural constraints refer to the determinants that hold people in patterns of interaction within groups, based on the interpretation of shared symbols, rituals and practices. Symbols of healthcare professions may include any of the artefacts that comprise practice, such as specific medical language, discourses and 'tools of the trade'. Rituals and practices may include client assessment, contributing specifically to specific client care, writing clinical notes, doing preventative, maintenance or remedial therapeutic work, and any of the habitual interactions that occur during these practices.

An example of specific medical language is: 'Mr Jones has circumoral cyanosis and dyspnoea'. Discourses are conversations and ways of speaking that convey the relative roles, intentions, status and authority of the speakers. An example of discourse is:

Nurse: Mr Jones has circumoral cyanosis and dyspnoea.
Doctor: Mr Jones has respiratory distress, sit him upright, give oxygen intranasally, and I'll be there stat.

(In this example, the nurse already knew the diagnosis, but did not state it, as that would be to assume a diagnostic role. She also had Mr Jones sitting upright, had made sure he was not alone, and had checked the orders to ensure oxygen prn was ordered and had begun therapy.)

'Tools of the trade' include all of the equipment and technologies used in practice, how they are used and by whom, to denote cultural norms. Tools of the trade in healthcare professions come in all sizes and include assessment forms, agency vehicles, infusion pumps, CAT scanners, dialysis machines, fob watches, suture scissors, uniforms, work shoes and identification tags. The public knows who works the equipment and technologies and assigns respect and deference according to the relative importance of these cultural symbols, rituals and practices. For example, greater deference is usually paid to the person operating the CAT scanner than it is to the person taking the client's temperature.

Rituals and practices form the fabric and culture of daily work and they are plentiful. For example, it may be part of healthcare professionals' cultures to wear a uniform at work. A uniform serves many purposes and maintains a predictable pattern of interpersonal relating. It is a symbol of service and servitude and lets everyone know where the professional fits in the order of the organization. Doctors do not generally wear uniforms; usually they wear a white coat and they drape a stethoscope around their necks, even if they are not in the vicinity of clients. The symbolic representation of doctors' dress and the draped stethoscope tells people about their role and status in the healthcare organization. When other healthcare professionals in hospitals started draping stethoscopes around their necks, it violated the cultural norm of 'white coat and stethoscope equals doctor'. Similarly, when nurses stopped wearing veils, bonnets, aprons and stripes on their lapels, some clients and medical and allied staff bemoaned the lack of identification and hinted at possible drops in standards as the cultural fabric of the organization unravelled.

Over time, cultural expectations are shifting to accommodate changes, not only in practitioners' dress, but also in their role relationships with other staff. For example, in some organizations, nurses and midwives no longer rush to greet doctors, nor carry their files, nor set up for minor surgical procedures in units, nor rush after them to request written orders, nor accede to an unwritten cultural convention that doctors are 'godlike' and beyond question and reproof. However, in other organizations, and at an individual level, cultural conventions of subservience and deference beyond the reasonable bounds of adult–adult communication still control the ways in which practitioners relate to one another. Even though cultural constraints may seem to be relatively insignificant in themselves, they are nevertheless very powerful, because they represent shared symbols, rituals and practices that have endured over time as unquestioned assumptions of authority, status and ways of communicating. Therefore, healthcare professionals who choose to operate outside the unwritten rules of cultural constraints may find themselves censored and chastised by individuals and the organization to varying degrees.

Reflector

What other examples of cultural constraints can you imagine? If you are having trouble getting started, think about the kind of symbols, rituals, habits and practices that are unquestioned in your workplace, that do not seem to have any reasonable basis, other than that they have endured for some time and define the ways people relate to one another.

Economic constraints

Economic constraints refer to a lack of money and the resources money can provide. If you have been practising for some time, you are most probably conversant with this constraint and have plenty of examples of it. Money, or lack of it, drives contemporary healthcare. Each year the 'bad news' about health organization budgets is circulated: financial belts are tightened further, resources are cut, organizations are closed down or downsized, experienced people are offered voluntary redundancy packages, staff–client ratios suffer or are rationalized by budgetary constraints, and profits are favoured over people – or so it seems for many workplaces.

No constraint exists alone. For example, economic constraints flow out of and into other constraints. A scenario reads like this:

> Statement: The budget looks bleak for next year. Positions must be cut. A new education role had been projected for next year, but it will need to go 'on hold'.
>
> Question: Who would have occupied that education role?
>
> Answer: An experienced diabetes educator.
>
> Question: But how does this decision sit with the acquisition of a new CAT scanner next year worth the salary of three diabetes educator positions?

In this scenario, cultural and economic constraints combine to compete for precious resources.

Reflector

What group of people generally win in the competition for economic resources in your workplace? Why?

Not all economic constraints operate at large levels. They may start at local levels with familiar places and faces and eventually balloon out into far bigger, faceless forums. For example, consider an everyday issue as simple as the allocation of staff by their peers to wards and units to cover work requirements adequately. In this scenario, the professionals 'control' the allocation of resources within their budget, and they have the responsibility to ensure that healthcare contexts are staffed adequately. However, the managers are given finite resources, and they are in turn constrained by bosses up the line in the hierarchy, who in turn may ultimately place the blame for poor staff ratios on the government's health budget. In this manner we perpetuate the blame shifting exercise of 'It is not my fault, it is someone else's fault.' So when healthcare professionals leave their careers to become shopkeepers or drug reps and care agencies and national governments bemoan the lack of qualified healthcare staff, who stands up to expose economic constraints and poor staff ratios, which caused overworked, underpaid professionals to fall out of enchantment with their practice, because they could bear the constraints no longer?

Reflective practice uncovers the nature and effects of economic constraints and attempts to locate associated constraints, which may or may not be conducive to change. This is not to claim that the reflection alone will fix a budgetary cut, or convince a health minister to leave open a cost-ineffective hospital. No grand claims such as these can be made for reflection, but it can throw a light on economic tendencies and patterns and identify reactions of organizations to financial strictures in the system. Having located these, concerted reflection and strategies can put into place a means by which economic constraints can be challenged through individual and collective political action at local, state and federal levels. The type of reflection in this book best suited to tackle such an overt political agenda is emancipatory reflection, because it identifies and challenges all of the constraints that work against effective healthcare.

Historical constraints

Historical constraints are those factors that have been inherited in a setting, which remain unquestioned because of the precedence of time and convention. History creates the present and hints as to the possible nature of the future. This is not to suggest that history is immutable and that once set in place historical events cannot be diverted, adapted or ceased from their original trajectories. Rather, it has been said often that if we are ignorant of our past, we are helpless to identify our present and to shape our future. History is important, because it helps us to see what has been, in order to decide on what can be.

In healthcare practice, historical precedents align themselves closely with cultural and social determinants. In other words, the cultural norms created by symbols, rituals and practices combine easily with the interpersonal relationships defined by social contexts, to become relatively enduring events and behaviours, because of the influence of strong historical antecedents. Even so, trends can be disrupted, stalled and/or reversed depending on what forces win in the powerful stakes of creating history.

For example, historical records inform us that the first officially recognized midwives were wise women, who cared for women giving birth. The practice of midwifery continued unaffected until the Middle Ages, when it received negative attention from the male-dominated state and the Church, at the time of the witch-hunts in Europe, which lasted from the fourteenth to the seventeenth centuries (McCool and McCool 1989). The midwives of that time worked with herbs and other healing modalities. The first regulation of their practice came about because of fear of their powers as lay healers and their supposed identity as witches, together with the political and religious threat they posed to the dominant forces, by virtue of being self-directed and influential women (Ehrenreich and English 1973; Kitzinger 1991). It is not surprising to find that the extermination of midwives as witches came at a time when medicine was reaching its peak.

Midwifery history does not provide a clear description of the connections between midwives and witchcraft (Oakley and Houd 1990). While there is no proof that midwives were also witches, many women were sacrificed to the ideals of the Church and the state, which combined forces to eradicate the 'evil' of the time. However, it has been deduced that the terms 'woman', 'witch', 'midwife' and 'wise woman' were used interchangeably, and that these people all fell within the category of 'a great multitude of ignorant persons' (Oakley and Houd 1990: 25–6).

The witch-hunts and the rise of medicine are considered to be the two main reasons why midwives' practice became more and more regulated. From a beginning of autonomous practice in the care of mothers and babies, midwives became subordinated to the medical model as 'obstetric nurses'. It is interesting, however, that the first men involved in the care of women giving birth were barber surgeons, who were called in by the midwives to perform destructive surgery on obstructed dead foetuses. It was not until the seventeenth century, when forceps were developed, that barber surgeons were present to assist in live births (Kitzinger 1991). As women were excluded from education, the barber surgeons and the physicians were men, and thus the male domination of midwifery was set into train.

This small slice of midwifery history informs us about some of the present-day struggles in which midwives find themselves. While being advocates of birth as a natural process, they nevertheless are aware of the problems that can occur in complicated cases, and they know they must accede to the knowledge and skills of staff better qualified to intervene when things go wrong. However, in remaining mothers' and families' advocates, midwives struggle to ensure that pregnancy and birth are natural processes in a culture that has historically looked at medical and surgical intervention to eradicate delays, discomfort, pain and unusual and potentially life-threatening circumstances. The problem for midwives is that biomedical arguments for intervention win out against 'being with' women in a natural process of waiting and supporting. Midwives know that it is historically, culturally and socially imprudent to question such arguments, so the intervention rates continue to rise in a well-intentioned, fear-based society.

History influences the present and shapes the future, but different people can perceive it differently and it can be rewritten according to the dominant values and voices of the time. Reflective practice allows healthcare professionals to examine the events of the past to better understand present-day practice and envision the kind of future they want for themselves and the people in their care. This is not to underestimate the power of historical constraints, as they are a force with which to reckon. Nevertheless, change is possible. Change can only come with awareness and action, so reflection is integral to practice improvements, as historical constraints are recognized and worked on systematically, through reflective processes oriented to action and change.

Political constraints

Political constraints are about the power, competition and contention in relationships in day-to-day life. Politics is everywhere, not just in parliaments and courthouses. The early feminist movement had a catch-cry: 'The personal is political'. This statement brought home the message that power and power-plays are inherent to everyday human life and that oppression and dominance are ever-possible states of human existence; they happen wherever and whenever people struggle for ascendancy and power. Any healthcare professional may use power against another healthcare professional and attempt to dominate the wishes and intentions of another person. Political issues do not have to be about big things, such as who wins an election, or sits on a powerful committee; political issues may be about who goes to lunch first and who influences the senior management in the dispensation of rewards and incentives.

Reflector

Reflect on the sources of political constraints in your work. To do this, think about who constrains you from being the healthcare professional you might ideally choose to be, when, how and why, with their power and influence.

Power is potent in organizations, because their structures and functions are conducive to the distribution of power through everyday practices, acted out through the authority of seniority and expertise in the 'pecking order' of the hierarchy. Proponents of organizational theory claim that organizations have changed over time. Organizational structures and processes have moved 'from the centralised control of bureaucracies' in the 1950s and 1960s 'to shared decision-making through consultation and participative management' in the 1970s and 1980s, to the 1990s' focus on 'best practice, customer-focused action and outcomes; and the manager's role as a researcher, teacher and enabler of creativity' (Anderson 1996: 30). Even so, practice stories convey themes of powerful domination and control by political forces and people in hospitals and healthcare agencies.

Power does not have to be a 'bad thing' – it can be a force for potentiating positive outcomes. The difficulty arises in the definition of positive and negative, as the question can be rightly asked: 'Positive or negative for whom, and why?' Power becomes one-sided and iniquitous when this question is not asked and the game of politics is played for the game itself. When politics constrains the ways in which people interact, it is not the reasonable, well-argued position that is heard and acted on, but rather the betraying voice whispered behind closed doors, or the powerful voice spoken loudly with the most authority and aggression. The nature of politics is power and contestation and that is how the game is played, but the game has rules and conventions to which appeals can be made for transparency and reasonableness.

Politics is alive and well in healthcare. The structure of healthcare organizations ensures the vivacity of politics and defines the ways in which interactions occur between individuals and groups competing for power, status and resources in the organization. Individuals engage in power-plays in clinical discourse and 'us and them' mentalities thrive where lack of understanding and respect for roles sets staff up against one another in a culture 'too busy and/or indifferent' to explore anything other than their own practice realities. For example, physiotherapists may not know or respect the roles of nurses; nurses may not know or respect the roles of occupational therapists or social workers, and so on. It takes time, effort and courage to break down political constraints. Reflective practice offers a means by which perceptions can be challenged, politics can be exposed and there can be some negotiation of political differences in the light of new information and a spirit of cooperation. This is not to underestimate the power of political constraints, because the powerful benefit from their powerful positions and are unlikely to give up the benefits of their power easily. In some cases, political constraints hold strongly against all attempts to appeal to them but, at the very least, reflective practice assists you in exposing and finding a voice to speak out against political injustices at work.

Social constraints

Social constraints are the habitual features of a setting and the ways in which people define themselves through interactions in that setting. They relate to interpersonal interactions and are connected closely to cultural and historical constraints, which are also seated in human interaction through shared meanings over time. The social norms of a setting vary – for example, the way you behave in the social setting of work is different to how your behave in the privacy of your own home. The way a midwife behaves in a birthing room may be different from the way they behave when receiving a baby from a Caesarean section. A physiotherapist may act in a certain way in a rehabilitative unit and another way in an intensive care setting. The point is that the social setting in some way determines the way we act and how we relate to other people within that setting.

Healthcare professionals may be most comfortable interacting within their own practice groups. The reasons are not difficult to speculate – individuals belonging to the same group are aware of the social conventions that govern their behaviour and they can embody them well and with relative ease. When we relate socially outside our preferred groups we need to be aware of acceptable ways of relating, so effective communication is maximized and misadventures are minimized. Confusion, misunderstanding and varying degrees of miscommunication are possible if we do not know how to relate to relatively unfamiliar individuals and groups. Healthcare professionals overcome social blunders and consequent negative outcomes by learning how to fit within the social setting of the workplace, and to interact appropriately with the people working there. Reflection facilitates learning, so that socially appropriate behaviours can be identified and practised.

Social constraints define relationships at work and assist us in acting appropriately, but they may also inhibit and limit our responses to a point where we hide behind appropriateness to save ourselves from closeness. For example, Jourard (1971) wrote about 'professional armour' and how health-care professionals can put on protective behaviours to shield themselves from the relative tragedies and uncertainties of daily practice. Professionals may also choose to limit the ways in which they show their thoughts and feelings to people in their care, so that they remain detached and aloof, risking little in social engagement with others at work. Reflective practice allows you to explore the ways you relate to others and to examine the reasons why and how social constraints may have developed your patterns of behaving that are sometimes non-productive.

Personal constraints

Personal constraints have to do with unique features about you as a person, shaped by influences in your life, into which you may or may not have insights. That is to say, you are as you are, but you may not know who and how you are. I have put this constraint last, because it is usually the first one health-care professionals think of when they are reflecting on their practice. In other words, I do not want to give it the same importance in this list of constraints, because I contend that we are not the main or sole reason things can 'go wrong' at work. While accepting that we may be in part responsible for some things some of the time, we nevertheless need to recognize the other con-straints that operate at work and elsewhere in our lives.

Personal constraints come about because of identified or unidentified obs-tacles inherent in the way we present ourself to the world and lead our own inner life with ourself. Self-work is personal work and it takes time, effort and courage to face yourself honestly, to identify strengths and weaknesses. In my opinion (Taylor 2000), and in the writing of other authors (Freshwater 2002a, 2002b; Johns 2002) healthcare professionals are all the more effective when they are actively and constantly working on reaching deeper levels of self-knowledge through self-developing processes, such as reflection, contempla-tion, meditation, visualization, prayer and thoughtful engagement in the arts, such as music, painting and poetry, and with other people in authentic communication.

Another way of looking at personal constraints in healthcare is to consider the deficits that you may be carrying in practice knowledge and skills. In other words, we have to face up to the fact that some professionals may have inadequate, outdated or incorrect knowledge and skills and these deficits could be constraining them personally from effective practice. Sometimes we are aware of what we do not know and we can take steps to amend this problem. Other times we may go along quite happily not knowing we have knowledge and skill deficits, until a 'near miss' happens and someone suffers at our hands. Everyone can make mistakes, and mistakes happen to the best people, but there is a big difference between mistakes and misadventures in practice, when the latter are brought about from knowledge and skill deficits. In this book, the type of reflection best suited to attending to this form of personal constraint is technical reflection, because it asks what is wrong or lacking and sets up a systematic means of questioning to arrive at solutions to clinical issues.

Summary

This section described cultural, economic, historical, political, social and personal constraints at work and the ways in which they may affect your practice. Looking at your own practice in order to raise your awareness about your own values and actions encourages you to shift your focus outwards towards the context in which you work and how you interact there. When you shift the focus away from blaming yourself exclusively, to reflect on cultural, economic, historical, political and social constraints issues that may be affecting your practice, you begin to see that that your work is complex and there are many reasons why things go wrong, and ways in which constraints may be identified, explored and changed. This book will help you to work through this reflective process with the aim of enlivening and enhancing your practice. Reflective practice is not a panacea for all the ills of your particular healthcare profession, but it provides a systematic process through which constraints can be identified and issues can be examined.

Ensuring quality practice through reflective processes

This section describes the means by which healthcare professionals can incorporate reflective processes into approved approaches for ensuring quality care. I suggest that quality care lies within practice in the therapeutic nature of caring relationships and that these can be uncovered and 'counted' as influential in the delivery of quality care to clients.

In the course of their daily work, healthcare professionals deal with issues which challenge the easy flow of events, by disrupting therapeutic relationships and outcomes. Reflective processes allow healthcare professionals to identify work issues and make the necessary changes to eradicate the disruptions and enhance therapeutic outcomes. Some issues healthcare professionals encounter in their work are described in this section.

Recognizing quality care

In healthcare systems, we tend to rely on numerical measures to identify quality care, by collating and analysing clinical indicators of excellence, which are observable and measurable. Quality care is in turn connected to evidence-based practice, in which it can be demonstrated that practice is being directed by the latest and best research findings. Evidence-based practice encourages observable and measurable assessment of quality care through quantitative means. Quantification relates to numerical assessment methods that give clinicians, managers and researchers statistical certainty that the best care outcomes are known, reliable and predictable, given standard, stable conditions in the clinical setting and adherence to proven procedures.

Most clinical indicators in which we have placed our faith to date have been verified as successful by quantifiable means, such as reduced infection rates, reduced length of stay in hospital, reduced readmission rates, high client satisfaction scores and so on. These means have relied mainly on numbers. Reflective practice requires linguistic processes, in the form of words, sentences, conversations, discourses and stories. How can reflective processes fit into a number-oriented system of quality assurance and evidence-based practice?

It requires a reconfiguration of what healthcare systems count as valuable, to incorporate clinicians' own insights into organizational policies and procedures, through in-depth analyses of their own practice. Reflective practice creates data capable of generating local theories of action that inform practice. Local theories are knowledge statements about practice that have been developed through focused attention on issues and problems, and the solutions thus generated have the capacity to be transferred to other similar situations, given that the insights and findings resonate with people working in those situations.

If reflective processes are to be valued as counting towards the assurance of quality care and best practice, they must be of a quality themselves as to assure effective outcomes. Another way of explaining this is that if you want to use reflective processes to make contributions to quality care where you work, make sure you are using them well yourself, so they have the best possible chance of being successful in guiding quality care that counts as best practice. This book coaches you in how to be effective in reflective processes. Once understood and practised, these processes have the potential to create a daily vigilance in you that keeps you alert to what is happening around you and increases the likelihood that you will be able to be active and enthusiastic about developing and maintaining quality care in your practice.

Often beyond the scrutiny of quantifiable indicators, there is an important aspect of quality care needing attention and acknowledgement in healthcare – that is, human-to-human relationships. The therapeutic nature of caring relationships within practice is inherent to practice and the quality of these caring relationships can be uncovered and 'counted' as important using reflective processes. This book guides you through three main types of reflection, which can assist you in identifying quality care, and/or instances of care needing improvement. Healthcare occurs in human settings where relationships are integral to the way care is given; therefore, systematic reflective processes enable healthcare professionals to enhance the quality of their work, for the benefit of their clients.

Recognizing work issues

After years of working with nurses and midwives to assist them in becoming reflective practitioners, I have noticed trends in the issues they face. After talking with other healthcare professionals, I suspect these issues are common to most practitioners, because they tell me about the difficulties in working together within healthcare organizations 'for the good of the client'. I present the main issues now and clarify them with reflectors, so you can see how they are part of everyday work and how they are rich sources for reflection and offer the potential for changed practice.

Engaging in self-blaming
When something goes wrong at work and you are at the centre of it, by making direct and simple connections between causes and effects you may decide that it is your fault and resort to self-blaming, guilt and self-recrimination. While there may be some occasions in which circumstances show that you have acted inappropriately or that you could have acted more wisely, there may also be occasions in which you have been too ready to blame yourself, by not being mindful of all the other constraints that were operating in the situation at that time. Reflective processes can alert you to ponder the determinants of situations and give you the means of working through them systematically so they can be managed now and prevented in the future.

Reflector
Do you engage in self-blame in your healthcare profession, or are you more likely to find fault with other people? Is there a midpoint between self-blame and blaming other people, and if there is, how can it be located?

Wanting to be perfect and invincible
Healthcare education gives the definite message to students that they are morally and legally responsible for competent and safe practice. To enforce the expectation, undergraduate programmes use examinations and essays to test knowledge acquisition and competency assessments for clinical skills. Healthcare professionals also learn, from the clinical areas in which they are placed

for experience, that the work demands high standards because people's health and welfare are at stake. We are not taught mediocrity in care, because we have to aim for the highest standards. Even so, mistakes happen because practice can be chaotic and complex and we do not always work carefully or effectively for various reasons. Mistakes can be costly, especially if they are related to certain risky aspects of care, such as the administration of drugs or the management of life-support systems.

Safe practice involves up-to-date knowledge and checks and measures for ensuring that mistakes are prevented, and it is part of responsible practice to pay due attention to these strategies. For fear of making mistakes, however, some healthcare professionals may develop ritualistic modes of behaviour, in which they act from a base of chronic anxiety to prevent mistakes from happening. In other words, a practitioner may think: 'If I always do this procedure, in this way, nothing bad will happen.' While this approach may produce safety standardization, it does not necessarily take account of other unexpected variables, such as how the client is responding.

Issues such as power, control and blaming other people may be manifestations of wanting to be perfect and invincible in all aspects of work. Versatility is needed in practice to deal with whatever comes up in the course of daily work. However, versatility can be mistaken for invincibility, and sometimes healthcare professionals may expect to 'walk on water', never being in trouble for making mistakes and wanting to cope magnificently in every situation.

Reflector

Do you have a need to be perfect in your work and to 'be all things to all people'? If you answered in the affirmative, you may need to look at the issue of your ideal need for perfection and invincibility.

Reflective processes encourage you to examine the reasons behind your need to be perfect and invincible, by asking yourself questions, such as how you came to feel that way, the purposes it serves, and why you continue to need to feel that way, even when it is not always possible or reasonable to reconcile that need to your work.

Examining daily habits and routines

Often, the most difficult things to change are those things that lie just in front of our noses, and are so commonplace that we cease to notice them, or to question their place in our lives. Work can be so commonplace that we take it for granted and never ask why we do what we do. Even though some work is anxiety-provoking, upbeat and high turnover, other aspects of work can be repetitive and tedious. Repetitive tasks can result in entrenched routines and habits that serve their purposes of getting the routine, essential work done, but can also become a source of practical and emotional boredom; as a result they become counterproductive as unexamined practices.

Daily habits and routines are a rich area for reflection, because they show you why you are practising in taken-for-granted ways and how you might be able to make some changes, given the constraints under which you work.

Reflector

Think about some of your work habits and routines. What are the benefits of these habits and routines and what are their 'down sides'?

One of the problems in dealing with this issue is recognizing the commonplace aspects of your work as they may be relatively invisible to you, even though you engage in them daily. Pretend you are a visitor to the ward or unit in which you work, or better still that you come from another planet, and that you know nothing of the habits and routines there. Pay careful attention to the mundane aspects of your workplace, such as who comes and goes, why, when and how. You may begin to see many issues that could benefit from reflection, such as traffic flow, how many times people in your care are disturbed from their rest, mealtimes, the timing of procedures, how staff and visitors relate to one another, who talks the most in interactions, why, with whom, with what authority, and with what outcomes, and so on. The possibilities are as bountiful as your willingness to observe and identify them.

Struggling to be assertive

There are many people interacting in healthcare settings, doing important work, most probably in a hurry, and with too few resources, so it is unsurprising that communication can become difficult. Add to this the cultural, social and historical constraints and the complexity increases. Then imagine particular circumstances when power is involved, such as when a person with greater power and authority is communicating with a person with perceived lesser status in the organization, and you have the right mix of constraints and conditions for one-way communication in which some people's voices are never or seldom heard. If the situation is to be challenged, someone has to find the courage to speak up and be assertive.

Reflector

Do you sometimes struggle to be assertive in your work? With whom are you most likely to lack assertion? Why?

Healthcare professionals need to be assertive in their communication, in order to be effective as clinicians, and to put forward the interests of their clients and their discipline in the interdisciplinary health team. If you are struggling to be assertive, you may be experiencing the effects of not 'finding your voice' at work, leading to feelings of frustration, or even powerlessness and apathy. The remedy may not be as simple as assertiveness training. You may also need to explore whether your lack of assertion is due to being silenced at work by powerful constraints that could make 'the world's best communicator' mute. Reflective processes assist you to identify constraints that have acted as silencing factors and you can begin to take steps to lessen, and eventually be freed from them.

Struggling to be an advocate
Advocacy means speaking up on someone else's behalf. Healthcare professionals need to speak up on behalf of people in their care and sometimes for themselves, especially when power relationships are at play – for example, for clients when medical language is too complex for them to comprehend. Hospital and clinic work situations may provide scant opportunities for clients to feel they can speak up for themselves, especially if other people with higher status seem to be too busy, unapproachable, too difficult to understand or unwilling to communicate at the level and rate the other person needs.

Reflective processes can help you understand why advocacy is difficult for you in relation to the constraints within which you are working. You may find that being an advocate has deeper foundations than you first imagined. Speaking up for someone else takes communicative skill, which is nurtured through experience and practised through confidence, both of which take time, effort and courage to develop. Although becoming an effective advocate is not a simple undertaking, it is possible through focused reflective processes.

Differentiating between ideal and real practice expectations
You need to be aware of the difference between ideal and real practice, because they are different, and the distinction can be the basis of recognizing issues in practice. We develop ideals through forming a value system. Values are what we hold as good, true and dear in our lives. For example, I value telling the truth, respect for others and being kind to other people. My values come from various sources, such as my family, friends, school, church, education and so on. My practice as an academic shows some or all of my values, because these form, and to some extent dictate, who I am and how I represent myself in the world. I can maintain my value system in most human interactions and in that sense I am 'true to myself'. However, sometimes I act outside my value system and the ideals I espouse may need to be altered or dropped to fit a given situation. For example, when I am trying to save someone else's feelings I do not always tell the whole truth, I do not respect people who abuse other people and sometimes I am too dammed angry to be kind to some people! In making these alterations to my espoused value system I have found instances in which my ideals do not always hold for me and I am clear in my own mind why I have made these value adjustments.

Reflective practice can assist you to see what parts of your work are based on ideals, and whether they are realizable in the face of work constraints. You may discover that your daily practice falls short of your ideals, and that this is not always a 'bad thing'. For example, if you think that, ideally, 'all people are good', you may be challenged when you are involved in healthcare interactions with people such as clients, families and other healthcare workers who have motives that do not fit your definition of 'good'. Even in the face of blatant contradictions of your ideals, you may try to hang on to them, to preserve some sense of personal integrity. When personal ideals are shattered in practice you may experience emotions such as loss, anger, confusion, help-lessness, lack of self-esteem, loss of sense of purpose and so on. Therefore, by reflecting on the issue of ideal versus real practice, you may be able to identify the origins of your firmly held values and explore whether they still serve you in every case in your work. You may need to reconcile the absoluteness of some of your ideals at work with relative considerations, while maintaining basic principles that guide your daily interactions with other people.

Reflector

Think of a personal value you hold dear in your work. Now, think of an instance in your practice when you were unable to hold on to that value. Why did you choose to act against your personal value and ideal practice?

Negotiating interprofessional boundaries

Healthcare professionals in organizations such as hospitals, clinics and profes-sional rooms need to work together as part of an interdisciplinary health team. To do this well, there needs to be a well developed sense of respect between practitioners for the work they do with clients. This respect assumes a sound level of knowledge about the other professionals' roles and responsibilities and how to work together at interprofessional boundaries.

Healthcare professions safeguard the scope, conduct and boundaries of their practices through codes of practice and codes of ethics. Codes of practice define the boundaries of practice activities, such as policies and procedures, and the expectations the community can rightfully hold in relation to that profession. Professional standards are derived from a profession's codes of practice and they are the means by which a profession is judged in cases where it is suspected that care has fallen below an acceptable clinical level. These professional standards also inform other healthcare professionals about the processes and procedures a profession is legally able to perform as accredited or registered practitioners. When another healthcare profession steps across the interprofessional boundary clinically, it is acting outside the legal parameters and clinical standards approved for that profession. For example, a registered nurse cannot diagnose, prescribe or provide medical intervention, and a social worker cannot perform surgery.

Codes of ethics give the parameters of moral rights and responsibilities for a profession. These codes describe the values of a profession and guide practitioners in making sound moral judgements about the issues that arise within their field of expertise. Many of these values, such as honesty, trust beneficence, non-maleficence and confidentiality, are shared by healthcare practitioners from other disciplines, as they agree that these values are foundational to ethical conduct in healthcare. Problems arise when there are moral issues across professional boundaries, which are interpreted differently, and/or when a practitioner acts outside the guidelines of their own moral code. For example, interprofessional boundaries may be tested when professions are competing for scarce healthcare resources, or when exclusive judgements need to be made about which client receives specialized care (e.g. a heart or liver transplantation).

Reflector

What legal and moral issues are there across your interprofessional boundaries? How are these issues managed?

Managing collegial relations

Relations between colleagues in healthcare settings can lack joy and friendship, and reasonably happy relations can sour and deteriorate due to all kinds of unexamined issues, such as lack of acknowledgement, jealousy, lack of sharing of knowledge and expertise, and that old-time 'evergreen', 'horizontal violence'. Many collegial issues are self-evident, as some colleagues may be only too willing to let you know, in no uncertain terms, just what irks them about you. At other times, you may get the sinking feeling that all is not well – there is less eye contact, less congeniality, unspoken rivalry and non-verbal messages, the meaning of which you can't quite discern.

Bullying can occur wherever people congregate and work in large numbers together, such as in schools, factories, businesses and organizations. Bullying, described specifically as 'horizontal violence' (Duffy 1995; Glass 1997), means a lashing outward, laterally against one's own group, and it is often associated with the need to overpower and subordinate others. It is often seen where people are working upwards through a hierarchical system and instead of remembering their early experiences and being empathetic towards others coming 'upwards', they use their increased seniority to 'give as good as they have been given' and perpetuate the culture of retribution and violence.

Reflector

Are you aware of issues of bullying and abuse in your healthcare profession? Who are the perpetrators and victims? What, if anything, is done about it?

Reflective processes can help in any difficult situation, because their first requirement is that you take time to think. Reflection does not promise to make your workplace a nirvana so everyone works together in harmony, or to alter anyone else's behaviour, but it can give you insights into why people behave as they do, and help you to reflect on ways to manage that behaviour. For example, the bullying behaviour may not happen in an instant; it may have been systematically and densely built up over years of unexamined intentions and unchallenged abusive acts. A perpetrator may develop abusive behaviour in a culture that allows horizontal violence to happen, and in a setting in which constraints cause healthcare professionals to act in dysfunctional ways towards one another. This insight does not condone the behaviour, rather it tries to deconstruct the context in which bullying is tolerated, to seek ways in which it can be challenged and possibly eradicated. This kind of reflective practice takes a great deal of thoughtfulness and courage, but nothing changes if we do not make it our business to change it.

Dealing with organizational and healthcare system problems
Organizational problems and changes in the healthcare system, such as staffing shortages, bed and ward closures, communication breakdowns, lack of acknowledgement and support from administration, downsizing and rationalization of services, and the introduction of new monitoring and management systems, such as case mix, diagnosis-related groups, quality assurance and competency standards, are just a few examples of the many and varied changes in healthcare organizations that are the result of shifts in the healthcare system at large. Most often, political and economic motives drive the changes.

As a healthcare professional, you may find that these problems impact on you and your work life directly in the form of increased workloads with reduced resources, and higher expectations that you will scale the career ladder, extend your qualifications, and enlarge your administrative and research output. While you are trying to adjust to these pressures, you may be receiving minimal support from other people, who may also be scrambling to keep their jobs and fulfil the sets of expectations imposed on them. All of these pressures and changes do not create cordial work relations, and communication within the organization can become distorted and exceedingly difficult to maintain at an effective level. This 'hotbed of discontent' is the very place in which reflective processes find their place, as they provide a systematic approach for making sense of how things came to be and how they could be different.

Managing self-esteem and worthiness problems
Self-esteem and a sense of worthiness may lie at the heart of many clinicians' concerns about themselves and their practice. Healthcare professionals are people and they, like other people, need to feel positive self-esteem and worthiness. Even though you may have been educated and prepared carefully for practice, you nevertheless remain human, first and foremost, with all the

foibles of humanness. Your humanness is at the same time your strength and vulnerability. The most qualified healthcare professional may seem self-sufficient and confident at work, but does that mean they do not seek approval from others, or need to be thanked for a job well done?

Your feelings of low self-esteem and unworthiness may spring from many causes and you will be the best person to identify what these are. Possibly, you may be feeling low self-esteem and unworthiness because no one has ever taken the time to thank you, to point out your strengths or to acknowledge you in any way at work. You may already know that you do not know everything, you cannot be everywhere, you cannot fix everything and it is not possible to be loved by everyone, but these realizations do not stop you from trying to be 'super professional'.

The problems of low self-esteem and a sense of unworthiness are so large that they lie at the basis of a happy life generally, not just work life. Sensing the immensity of these issues, I have made them the first step on the pathway to becoming a reflective practitioner. You will find that the first reflective task is to think about yourself and your rules for life, to gain a richer sense of who you are and what motivates you to be a healthcare professional. Although this first step may not solve all your feelings of low self-esteem and unworthiness, it will alert you to their presence and assist you in getting started on the process of building a positive sense of personal and professional worth.

Summary

This chapter introduced you to the nature of reflection and practice by covering definitions and sources of reflection, and literature pertaining to reflective practice in healthcare professions. The chapter also discussed the nature of caring in health professions, by responding to the questions: What is caring?, What is professionalized caring? Why do professionals care? Even though healthcare professionals may espouse caring values, it is not always easy to deliver quality care, so this chapter described the nature of professional work constraints and issues and suggested that, even against the difficulties, it is still possible to ensure quality practice through reflective processes.

Welcome to reflection! I hope that it will be positive, life-changing experience, even when it becomes challenging and you wonder why you decided to live a reflective life.

Key points

- Reflection is the throwing back of thoughts and memories, in cognitive acts such as thinking, contemplation, meditation and any other form of attentive consideration, in order to make sense of them, and to make contextually appropriate changes if they are required.

- Donald Schön emphasized the idea that reflection is a way in which professionals can bridge the theory–practice gap, based on the potential of reflection to uncover knowledge in and on action.
- Technical reflection, based on the scientific method and rational, deductive thinking, allows you to generate and validate empirical knowledge through rigorous means, so that you can be assured that work procedures are based on scientific reasoning.
- Practical reflection leads to interpretation for description and explanation of human interaction in social existence, and improves the way you communicate with other people at work, thereby improving your practice enjoyment and outcomes.
- Emancipatory reflection provides a systematic questioning process to help you to locate the bases of the problem, identify the political constraints and begin to address the issues, either alone or through collaborative action with other healthcare professionals.
- Healthcare professions are person-focused, helping professions requiring hard work and a strong knowledge and skill base from which to face the daily challenges of practice; therefore, systematic approaches to reflection and action are needed.
- Cultural, economic, historical, political, social and personal constraints may affect the ways in which you are able to interpret and act at any given moment at work.
- Cultural constraints refer to the determinants that hold people in patterns of interaction within groups, based on the interpretation of shared symbols, rituals and practices.
- Economic constraints refer to workplace issues caused by a lack of money and the resources money can provide.
- Historical constraints are those factors that have been inherited in a setting, which remain unquestioned because of the precedents of time and convention.
- Political constraints are about the power, competition and contention in relationships in day-to-day life and work.
- Social constraints are the habitual features of a setting and the ways in which people define themselves through interactions in that setting.
- Personal constraints have to do with unique features about you as a person, shaped by influences in your life, into which you may or may not have insights.
- When you shift the focus away from blaming yourself exclusively to reflect on cultural, economic, historical, political and social constraints that may be affecting your practice, you begin to see that

your work is complex and there are many reasons why things go wrong, and ways in which constraints may be identified, explored and changed.

- Issues faced by healthcare professionals that may benefit from reflection include engaging in self-blaming, wanting to be perfect and invincible, examining daily habits and routines, struggling to be assertive, struggling to be an advocate, differentiating between ideal and real practice expectations, negotiating interprofessional boundaries, managing collegial relations, dealing with organizational and healthcare system problems, and managing self-esteem and worthiness problems.

- Understood and practised, reflective processes have the potential to create a daily vigilance that keeps you alert to what is happening around you, and increases the likelihood that you will be able to be active and enthusiastic about developing and maintaining quality care in your practice.

2 Preparing for reflection and the REFLECT model

Introduction

In this chapter I describe qualities and hints for reflecting, and guide you through your first systematic reflective task, so that you can experience reflective processes first hand. I also describe the role of a critical friend, to help you to reflect at deeper levels, and I explain that this is a role you can adopt in helping others to become more effective in their reflective practice. Finally, I describe the 'Taylor model of reflection', using the mnemonic device REFLECT, to give you an approach that is easy to remember and apply to systematic reflection in your work.

Qualities for reflecting

After years of practising, teaching and researching reflection, I have come to the conclusion that it takes considerable time, effort, determination, courage and humour to initiate and maintain effective reflection.

Taking and making the time

Reflection requires time and that is one of the main reasons why healthcare professionals do not make a commitment to creating a reflective work life. I imagine that you are a busy person already, most probably working shifts or long days, managing home life to keep up to family responsibilities, and trying to fit in some personal fun, leisure and relaxation when you can. This means that you may be hesitant to squeeze in any more activities, such as taking or making time to reflect on your practice. Therefore, the first quality you need to have as a successful reflective practitioner is the willingness to take and make time in your life to make a commitment to the process. Only you can take and make the time for reflecting. When you experience the benefits of reflective practice, you may be keen to continue, so when you do take and make the time to reflect, give it your full attention to do it well, to maximize the potential for its success.

Making the effort

Life is full of activities, few of which happen if you do not make an effort, which you will make when you suspect that something is of value, reasonably easy and of benefit to you personally. Reflective practice is all of these things – worthwhile, easy and beneficial. However, if you are new to reflective practice, you require some fundamental skills which will take some effort to acquire. This book guides you through all of the skills you need, but you have to make the effort to read the words, assimilate the information and maintain the practice. As your work life is inextricably connected to your personal life, by association, reflective practice means a commitment to yourself, which requires effort in creating and maintaining a healthy lifestyle, such as getting regular rest and exercise, healthy nutrition, stress management and maintaining satisfying relationships with your family and friends. It is entirely up to you to make the effort to be involved in your work and life and I commend regular reflection as an integral part of it, because it is really worth the effort.

Reflector

Do you have trouble making an effort to be involved in potentially useful activities? Why? In what ways can you ensure you make the effort to reflect?

Being determined

Determination is needed for reflection, because it is easy not to begin, or to stop regular reflective processes, due to tougher pressures that compete for your time and attention. It takes determination to get started and to keep going on reflection, because lack of resolve can easily result in inactivity, as reflection surrenders to other demands. The multifaceted demands of life will not cease, but you have the right to choose how and when you will respond to them. Determination will give you the power to propel your intentions forward into actions. Determination will also ensure that you keep on reflecting. Be determined!

Having courage

You need courage to look at yourself and your practice, because it takes honesty and frankness to move outside your comfort zones. It also takes courage to invest yourself in the depth of reflection needed to change dysfunctional procedures, interpersonal interactions and power relations at work. Work issues and problems become identified as such because they present dilemmas and are inherently difficult to face and solve. However, issue-identifiers and problem-solvers are not faint-hearted people; they are people prepared to muster and develop the courage needed to face up to and tackle difficulties directly. When you reflect intently on your work problems and issues, you need courage to identify constraints within your practice and workplace, and begin to make changes. You may find opposition from other people, who have political motives for maintaining the status quo, so they may try to betray you or display open aggression to change, and/or block any progress you may be making. Added to facing other people's reactions is the courage you require to face yourself. Reflective processes identify your own patterns of thinking and reacting, which may need adaptation. This is not to infer that all reflective practitioners have immense courage to always be proactive and assertive at work, because this is not necessarily the case. On the contrary, they are people who muster the courage to face the next step in the process, and having achieved that, move on to the next step. If you think of this as 'sequential courage', you may see that you are also capable of it.

Reflector

Think about your preparedness to reflect on your practice issues, in relation to the courage you might have to face them squarely. It might help to imagine any people or situations you find intimidating in some way, and ask yourself why they have power over you. When you have some tentative answers to those questions, imagine ways you could build your courage sequentially to reflect systematically on practice issues concerning the intimidation you are feeling.

Using humour

At this point, you may think that reflection is sounding very serious, complex and difficult, because it takes time, effort, determination and courage. Even though reflection needs to be approached seriously, and it has the potential to be complex and difficult, it is not always onerous and without some degree of fun. Healthcare professionals have a propensity for seeing the funny side of life and work, because humour is an effective way of lightening our workloads by making the day appear to go faster and easier. It also helps us to look less seriously at ourselves and other people. Reflection can incorporate humour by putting the memories of even the most gruelling challenges into perspective, and by naming the curious aspects of our work culture that have their absurdly funny side when viewed through that lens. Developing a mature sense of humour is an effective repellant for anxiety and it forms strong bonds with colleagues, who resonate with subtle messages within shared jokes or funny clinical stories. Reflection using humour provides an alternate source of insights into the nature of work constraints, because when they are 'turned on their heads' to intentionally look silly, cultural, economic, historical, political, social and personal constraints can lose some of their sting. Effective reflective practitioners demonstrate a sense of humour in the way they tackle their work and lead their lives, so be assured that reflection is not all serious; it can have its funny side.

Reflector

Imagine a practice situation in which you were feeling overwhelmed in some way and you wanted the 'floor to open up and swallow you'. Now stand back and look at yourself in that situation. Was there anything laughable about it? In hindsight, is there a lighter side that you can now see?

Summary

When you are ready to reflect and to maintain a reflective attitude to your life and work, you will most probably already possess many of the requisite qualities of taking and making time, making the effort, being determined, having courage and knowing how to use humour. These qualities will serve you well as you develop reflective knowledge and skills. Even if your levels of these qualities are low and almost imperceptible, they can be nurtured through reflective practice.

A kitbag of strategies

There are many strategies you can use when engaging in systematic reflection. Some inspire reflection, others guide, and some may inspire and guide you simultaneously. The following kitbag of strategies contains approaches that are like ingredients for a recipe and you should feel free to use and adapt them in any combinations and quantities you prefer. The kitbag suggests using reflective strategies such as writing, audiotaping, creating music, dancing, drawing, montage, painting, poetry, pottery, quilting, singing and videotaping. While this is not a finite list of reflective strategies, it is designed to help you get started and to have fun experimenting with a variety of methods.

Writing

When reflective processes are taught to people in practice, the impression is often given that keeping a journal or log of some sort is a fundamental requirement. Even though writing is an important means of recording your thoughts and feelings, it is not the only way of aiding and recording your reflection. This news may come as a pleasant surprise if you are someone who has trouble writing things down, or prefers other means of thinking systematically. Writing can be easy and effective and this section guides you in writing reflectively and creatively.

Reflector

If you have trouble writing, spend some time thinking about the possible reasons why. Do you associate writing with assessment of some kind? Do you imagine your writing may not compare well with other people's efforts? Write down the reasons why you might be having trouble writing, but write the ideas quickly in whatever form it takes to get them down on paper or the computer screen. Keep a copy of this and continue reading this section.

To prepare for writing, you need an exercise writing book or a computer or typewriter. Starting with handwriting materials, I suggest that you buy a fixed-page exercise book, so that you will be less likely to tear out pages when you are tempted to edit your writing. This may mean that your journal becomes 'messy', but it will be complete, 'warts and all'. Completeness is necessary so that you have a complete record of all your thoughts, especially if they change direction or move through unexpected areas. The pen, pencil or biro you use should handle well with minimal drag, so you can write quickly and easily. You might prefer to buy a special set of writing materials that encourage you to write and that you keep especially for reflection.

When you write don't be concerned about stylistic aspects, such as neatness, grammar, spelling and punctuation. The journal is yours, shared only as you choose, so there is no need to edit the writing for other people. The structure you use will be according to your growing expertise and confidence, and in the early part of your reflective experience this book guides you by posing questions and exercises to get you accustomed to what to write, when, how and why. When you reflect through writing, a particular mental approach is useful, such as spontaneity, openness and honesty, and these qualities are discussed later in this chapter.

If you are using a computer, you will most probably be aware of the usual tips for computing, such as making files, using good quality CDs or memory sticks, and saving your document often if you do not have an automatic save function. The best hints I can give you are what to avoid. Just type; don't edit your writing by cutting out sentences and paragraphs. Unlike word processing for formal tasks such as assignments, it is a good idea to type spontaneously as you think, without much, if any, planning. Thoughts may come in random order and themes may not be connected. This is the way some thinking happens privately, so don't try to change it or put it into a 'sanitized' form to suit a wider audience. Don't shift chunks of writing to other parts of the document to make it look better, or for it to be more grammatical or ordered.

If you are using a typewriter, it is also important for you not to try to order or edit your writing, so it looks nice or reads well. You need to let your typing flow with your thoughts and 'learn to live with' any disordered typing mess which may arise. You also need to keep anything you write in a self-holding folder, which keeps all the pages in the order in which they were typed.

Audiotaping

Not everyone is blessed with a love of writing and an ability to do it easily, and if you are such a person it may be good for you to learn that you can reflect without a lot of writing. If you are really systematic in how you use the other methods I'm suggesting here, you may be able to avoid writing altogether. Do you enjoy telling stories? If you do, you could tell your stories into a voice recorder so you have a record of what you say. Once you get over the awkwardness of sitting alone and chattering away to yourself and a machine, you will get accustomed to reflecting through talking. If you feel a bit silly at first, say it out loud, experience the feeling completely, and then choose to 'get over it'. Value the silent gaps which may also occur when you are drawing breaths or thinking quietly to yourself. Let the words come easily and effortlessly. Also, leave your words unedited by speaking unselfconsciously and by resisting the temptation to rewind and tape over certain sections.

If you are intending to use the voice recordings without any written notes to yourself, you need to develop the habit of reviewing what you said previously to record verbal remarks on successive recordings. In this way you will be able to keep a progressive record of the insights you have gained, so that you can make connections to what is yet to become apparent through the reflective process. This may mean that you accumulate a lot of audiotapes, so be sure to date and label them carefully, so you know which ones to replay as the need arises. The reflective processes described in this book work just as well by audiotaping as they do by writing, so long as you review the audiotapes frequently and carefully to identify and work on connections in what you have said about your practice. Alternatively, you may choose to make summary notes in a journal to complement your audiotapes, thereby tracking your reflective progress.

Reflector

Locate a voice recorder and record yourself talking about a happy childhood memory. After this, record yourself talking about why it was a happy occasion and why it still means so much to you. This exercise will give you some idea of whether taping your reflections will be useful for you.

Creative music

Have you noticed how music evokes emotions and memories? For example, music can make you sing, cry, laugh and open up to reminiscence. Playing personally significant music can heighten your awareness and put you into a reflective space. If this is the case for you, play music when you reflect and allow it to enhance your thinking processes.

Alternatively, you can 'make your own kind of music'. You do not have to be a musician to make music, if you simply let the instrument express how you are feeling and thinking. For example, you could beat out a rhythm on a drum or the back of a lid, shake a tambourine or a bag full of marbles, or strike randomly on a musical keyboard such as a piano, organ or xylophone. While you might make a fairly awful noise, that few musicians might call music, it is nevertheless important to make the sound. Let the volume and tempo of the notes express your feelings, loudly and quickly for anger, quietly and regularly for peacefulness, and so on. The creation of the music will help you to vent your feelings and to get in touch with your emotions, and this is helpful to get you into the mood for effective reflection.

If you have formal training and musical skills, you can create a more harmonious sound to inspire your reflection or to help you create sounds which represent what you are thinking. Thoughts and feelings are components of reflection and they can become locked in if they cannot find expression.

Play your music, or make your noise, and reflect on what is happening. You may find creative expression for feelings you are having about clinical issues and, as you are experiencing them, tune in to reflective insights. Once the stories start to flow through the release of music, you will have some substance on which to reflect and you can use music at any stage of the reflective process thereafter.

Dancing

You may claim that you are not a dancer, but if you have some means of mobility, you can dance. You do not have to be upright and bipedal to dance. People in wheelchairs and on walking aids can dance. Even if you feel like a baby elephant, or that you have two left feet when you try to dance, move your body anyway. It's easy if you just let go and dance, with or without music. Move by whatever means you have and let your body show you how you feel about work issues. At the same time, as with any other creative expression, you can also notice yourself as an interested observer. The feelings and thoughts evoked by dance will be useful for reflective processes. Having been evoked, thoughts and feelings can be channelled into the systematic reflective processes which are described in this book.

Record the reflections evoked or played out through dance. You could audio- or videotape the thoughts as partial or complete stories. A videotape is especially helpful, as it can capture the dance and your reflections during or after. The recording needs to be available for reviewing, so you can make progressive reflections as new issues emerge from your practice. If dancing inspires reflection or represents what you are thinking and feeling, it may be a creative reflection possibility for you.

Reflector

Dancing as a release is an interesting way of preparing yourself for reflection. Try dancing to a familiar tune. Do the music and the movement take you to another time and place? What memories and sensations does it conjure up for you?

Drawing

You may have the ability to draw what is in your head and 'heart', but if you do not, don't worry. Simply think of drawing as systematic doodling and you might feel a bit more confident about using it as a means of reflecting. Remember also that drawings are whatever you say they represent, so they do not need to be realistic or accurate, or to fulfil other artistic criteria. Whether the drawings happen spontaneously as an expression of what you are thinking and feeling, or whether they happen intentionally as a result of these processes, they can be useful with interpretations of your clinical experiences.

When you have drawn or doodled, record your responses to, or reasons for, the drawings you have made in relation to issues you are experiencing at work. Record your insights systematically in a lasting form so they can be revisited. For example, you could compile them in a book with space in between each for interpretations and insights, or you could record your reflections by speaking into a tape recorder. If you are keeping a journal they could be incorporated into what you are writing. Do whatever feels right for you.

Montage

A montage is a collection of images, often created from pictures, words and symbols cut out from old magazines and newspapers. If you have the time and interest in making a montage this may be an excellent way of assisting your reflective processes. As you search for images to express what you are thinking and feeling about clinical issues, you might find that you begin to reflect more fully, so that the emergent montage is a comprehensive representation of the sense you are making of certain practice events. On the other hand, the montage may provide you with a glimpse of where further reflection may take you, and you may not make connections until later when you take previous montages out of storage to review them.

Regardless of the way in which you organize your montage-assisted reflections, you need to record successive interpretations, so that the processes described in this book can be applied to them. The assimilated ideas and themes may be represented in other montages as you progress as a reflective practitioner and form a pictorial account of your personal and work insights.

Reflector

Collect some old magazines, scissors, glue and paper. Create a montage that depicts you as you see yourself now. When it is complete, take it to a friend and tell them about your montage, pointing out what the symbols and pictures mean to you. When you are ready, create a montage that depicts you as a practitioner and use a similar process to tell someone about your professional self. Invite that person to reciprocate and offer to listen to their account.

Painting

Watercolours, oils or acrylic paints can be used to paint a picture of your inner self and your practice. By painting, you can represent a situation, a thought, an outcome, or whatever it is that needs depiction for further thought. It does not matter if it turns out to be a mess, because you are the painter and your painting is what you say it is. Let's face it – your painting may not be up to gallery standard, but it will be valuable for you as it can depict your responses to issues in your practice. As you are painting, notice the colours you choose and how you apply the paint. Tune in to what you are thinking and feeling as you paint each stroke. You can paint spontaneously in response to your emotions and thoughts, or you can make deliberate strokes to create a painting to slow down and structure your thinking.

Keep all your paintings and a commentary about them on tape or in a journal. Issues change over time, and you may notice that your painting style changes with them. It is important that you make sense of your paintings and incorporate your interpretations into the systematic reflective processes described in this book. Use this method for as long as it is helpful, in combination with other methods, which provide some written or spoken words about the meaning of the paintings, where they fit, and why, in your reflective practitioner experiences.

Poetry

While making no claims to be Shakespeare, everyone can write poetry which has personal style and meaning. If you know the rules of poetry, by all means apply them, but even if you don't have the slightest idea of the structure of a poem, you could write one anyway. I write poetry from time to time and I imitate the rhythm and flow of other poems I have read, or I simply put as many words along one line as I fancy. My poems may never be published, but every time I take my own poetry book off the shelf and read it, my words bring back all the thoughts and feelings I had at the time of writing. This is why I think poetry could help you as you engage in systematic reflection on your practice.

When I write poetry I just let the words come. Sometimes the words repeat in my head until I can write them down. The slightest inspiration can be the basis of a poem. If you have had a hectic day at work, which has stirred up a lot of emotions and thoughts, try putting them into words. Your poem might be one line, or develop into proportions that would make Shakespeare envious. It does not matter, just let the poem flow as long as it needs to, so that you can express the issues on your mind.

As with all creative expressions for assisting reflection, you need to record your responses to your poetry, explaining when and how you wrote it, why and for whom, and what it means in relation to your practice reflections. Keep all your poems and commentaries and incorporate them into any other methods you are using for reflection.

Reflector

Imagine an event of any kind that happened to you within the last week or so. Write a short poem that begins with the first line: 'Last week I . . .' There is no limit to the words and lines in the poem – just let it flow.

Pottery

Based on the idea that anything is accessible to you if you can imagine it, pottery is another creative possibility to inspire and represent reflection. Not only is clay a wonderful medium for venting your emotions, it can form into many shapes, forms and symbols, which can represent clinical issues. If you have had a particularly terrible day at work why not throw the clay literally, for example, at the wall? Alternatively, you can play with clay or make works of art. It is up to you. If you create a clay form spontaneously or intentionally, notice how you are feeling and the thoughts you are having in relation to work. You might create a series of pots or pieces, and give them a name according to their evolution. Keep all the dried clay pieces, or take a photograph and record your insights successively to weave them into future reflections.

Quilting

Quilting is a deliberate act of sewing to represent selected themes of life. The symbols are selected carefully to contribute to the whole story depicted in the quilt. As you sit and sew, you can reflect on each symbol, and how it relates to the whole. In between quilting you can record your reflections with other methods for reflecting you may be using, such as writing or audiotaping.

Singing

You can sing by creating melodies and words that come spontaneously from a creative space inside yourself. As with many creative tasks, this can be difficult if you are overly self-conscious. To get started, sing a song you know. This will help you get used to the sound of your own singing voice. As you will be singing in private it does not matter if you sing off key or if your lyrics are less than poetic. Just open your mouth, breathe in, and sing out spontaneously!

As this is singing with reflective practice intentions, you need some form of recording, such as audiotaping or videotaping. You can decide on your level of comfort and skill in using either of these two recording methods. Also, you need to write successive interpretations of, and insights into, your songs and singing, noticing the words you used, the volume, pitch and mood of your singing, and your thoughts and feelings as you sang. These ideas and any more you develop along the way can be orchestrated into the other methods of reflection you are using, so that you can gain maximal effects from your reflective practice.

Videotaping

If you have ready access to video equipment, you might like to consider video-taping as the primary medium by which to enhance your reflection. One of the obvious benefits of using this medium is that you will be able to review yourself in terms of what you say and how you say it. Your own non-verbal cues may also be interesting for you to observe. For example, in telling some of your clinical stories, you may find that there is a substantial emotional component of which you were not fully aware. Your posture or pitch of voice may have something to tell you about yourself and the way a practice issue is affecting you. When you use the reflective processes described in this book, you will discover that they require you to be as honest and frank with yourself and your work as you can. Seeing yourself respond to these questions may enhance your reflections as you ask yourself about your non-verbal and verbal representation as portrayed on video.

As you need to make sense of your reflections, you need to develop a method for amassing progressive insights, questions and connections in your practice. You may choose to record these impressions directly on the video or into some other form of semi-permanent record, such as a journal or audiotape.

Reflector

Locate a video recorder and set it up so you can record yourself. Read the reflective exercise in this chapter. When you are ready, respond spontaneously to the questions on video.

Summary

Reflective processes include more than writing, which is good news for health-care professionals who have difficulty maintaining a journal. Reflection can also be inspired and maintained by creative strategies such as audiotaping, creating music, dancing, drawing, montage, painting, poetry, pottery, quilt-ing, singing and videotaping, used in any combination you prefer. In all of these cases, it is important to record reflections over time, so they can be analysed carefully for awareness and insights, and form a sequential account of your progress as a reflective practitioner.

Hints for reflecting

Before your first reflective practice exercise, there are some hints for reflect-ing that might also help relate to any strategies you might use to enhance reflection, such as writing, audiotaping, videotaping or some form of creative representation such as painting, montage, drawing, quilting, pottery, poetry, singing, dancing and/or creative music. In this section, I suggest that when you are reflecting you should remember to be spontaneous, express yourself freely, remain open to ideas, choose a time and place to suit you, be prepared personally and choose suitable reflective methods.

Be spontaneous

Be as spontaneous as possible in representing and recording your thoughts and feelings. It is from your frank and honest self that important insights come, from the depths of your emotions, where the meaning of motives and responses resides. Be spontaneous in your thinking, writing and other creative expressions, so that you create rich descriptions of your practice and your responses to issues and problems within it. If you are spontaneous you may uncover ideas and thoughts that have lain dormant for some time, or that you have kept locked away until 'some other time'. Be spontaneous in expressing all that you are now ready to express, and use the reflective guidelines in this book to help you make sense of it.

Express yourself freely

As your reflections are for yourself primarily, feel free to express them as dir-ectly and honestly as you can. These are *your* reflections, which you will only share with other people as you see fit, so be as explicit as you possibly can. This might mean that you swear sometimes, or use language in ways that you might not otherwise do in public. Sometimes a 'profanity' says all there is to say or write at that moment, and you can go back to it later to unpack what you actually meant when you said or wrote it. Admit to and face emotions and thoughts which emerge as you work through the reflective frameworks in this book. When you are expressing yourself freely, don't be slowed down and inhibited by trying to adhere to rules of grammar, spelling and punctuation. Just think, write, speak and so on, as freely as you can, so it pours out as directly and honestly as possible at that time.

Remain open to ideas

Reflection brings insights and partial 'truths' that may have some relevance for your practice. However, the first insight may not always be the best or the only flash of awareness that can enhance your work, so remain open to ideas so that they have a chance to grow, change or even disappear. Jumping to early conclusions may inhibit further insights and solutions, so be prepared for twists and turns in your thinking. Some questions may remain puzzles to which you always seek some answers, and that is OK, because sometimes what you learn in the search is more beneficial than what you find in the discovery. Enjoy the puzzles in reflective practice and realize that your answers will not be absolutes, but tentative responses to present problems and issues, that may need revisiting later.

Choose a time and place to suit you

Recognize the times of day when you feel alert and when you feel tired. Choose a time of day to reflect when you feel fresh and ready to give some quality time to thinking about your practice. Good planning will also mean that you set time aside in your busy life for reflecting; if it is not left to chance, it may mean that you are more likely to develop regular reflective habits. In this way, you create a time in which you can reflect, where no other pressures intervene for a while. Also, find a place to reflect that is conducive to thinking and creativity. If you are using creative strategies such as videotaping, creating music, dancing, drawing, montage, painting, poetry, pottery and quilting, these activities will to some extent determine the place in which you reflect. Even so, you can be creative in choosing places to reflect, such as parks, the beach, pool patios, aeroplanes, cruise ships and so on. The main requirement is that the place is conducive. Choose carefully a time and place in which to reflect and your reflections will be enjoyable and beneficial, while you also reward yourself by creating a space outside the confines and responsibilities of everyday work and life.

Be prepared personally

Identify the aspects of your lifestyle that put you in the best sense of freshness and preparedness. I have linked the two aspects because they relate to one another; if I feel fresh, I feel prepared for the activities of life, such as work, home duties, relationships and so on. Getting ready for reflection requires some personal preparation. What you do will be entirely up to you, but I suggest that to feel as fresh and alert as possible, you might like to do some favoured activities, such as walking, swimming, gym exercises, meditation, visualization or any other form of stimulation or relaxation which puts you into an attentive, imaginative mood.

Choose suitable reflective methods

Any of the methods/strategies in the kitbag discussed earlier, or whatever you imagine beyond the kitbag, may be used alone or in combination to enhance and maintain your reflective practice. All you have to do is decide what you want to do and set it into action. Choose your most favoured activities and experiment after that. For example, you may start by writing in a journal and then become more adventurous with video and dance. If you don't take it too seriously and have fun in the process, who knows what strategies you will use! The idea is to reflect as freely, spontaneously, deeply and honestly as possible, so experiment until you find the combination of methods which suit you best. Regardless of the reflective strategies you choose, you need to keep a record of your practice stories for reviewing, so be sure to build recorded summaries and insights into your chosen strategies.

Summary

When you reflect, by whatever method(s), it is important to consider how you prepare yourself and undertake the process. Remember to be spontaneous, express yourself freely, remain open to ideas, choose a time and place to suit you, be prepared personally, and choose suitable reflective methods: the rest will be fun and of benefit to you.

A reflective exercise

In this section I suggest how you can recall and record your childhood memories in relation to who you are now as an adult and a clinician. I guide you through a reflective exercise, in which you respond to structured questions. This exercise is to demonstrate reflective questions and responses. This is not to suggest that you are not already reflective, because you have managed your life to this point and much of that success has come about through your reflective ability. However, for some readers, this reflective exercise marks the beginning of their intentional and systematic reflection as a clinician. If this is the case for you, welcome to reflective practice and may it make you a happier and more effective person and clinician.

I invite you to use whatever method of reflecting you choose, such as writing, audiotaping or other creative ways of enhancing reflection as described in this chapter, to think about this exercise. You may find that the answers to some questions come quickly, while others need more time. Life is not always about happy memories either, and you may find that these questions bring up memories which may be tinged with sadness or some other emotion you have not faced before.

This is a good point in the process to make a comment about the *depth* of reflection. It is a good idea to reflect only to the level at which you are relatively comfortable. This does not mean that you avoid challenges surrounding unfinished issues, but that you choose to look at them at the rate and depth at which you feel able to cope. This is not a process of deep psychoanalysis, because you need a skilled person to guide you in deep personal exploration. What is being encouraged here is your willingness to be open to the questions and to respond to them as directly and honestly as you can.

Reflector

Think about the person you were as a child. Find a time in your childhood in which you felt you had a good sense of who you were. Record in writing, verbally or by some other creative representation, some spontaneous responses to the questions posed below.

What were you like as a child, physically, mentally, emotionally and spiritually?
Where did you live and what was it like?
Who were the important people in your life? Why were these people important to you?
What other influences were important in your childhood, such as other people, places and events?
What were some of the 'rules for living' you learned from these people, places and events?

Now that you have created a cameo of yourself as a child, make some connections to your adult work life as a healthcare professional, by responding freely to these questions.

Why did you want to become a healthcare professional?
Who were some of the important people in your life during your professional education?
What is important now in your practice and the ways you choose to work?

What, if any, childhood 'rules for living' have been transferred into your adult work life as a healthcare professional?

From your responses to these questions you may be able to see a little more clearly who you are as a person and a practitioner, and how you think your healthcare profession should be practised according to your personal values and ideals. Your responses may tell you a little or a lot about how you think your life and work should be conducted according to some of your personal ideals. The responses may also serve to show you how values, beliefs and actions can operate between the ideal expectations of childhood and the real experiences of adulthood. Keep your responses to this reflective exercise, so that you can identify connections in the stories you are yet to record. It is amazing how ideas fall into place when you take time to review them and put them into perspective. If you would like to take this exercise further, share your responses with a trusted friend, or offer some of them as a story to colleagues during a work break. You will find that you keep thinking about these questions and that other possible responses come to mind from time to time. Record all future responses to these questions and reflect on the additions, changes and extensions to your original thoughts. There is no end to reflection; it keeps on changing and moving forward.

Author's reflection

As a teacher, I usually try to undertake the tasks I construct for students, so I am happy to share with you how I have responded to this reflector.

I was born in Burnie, Tasmania, on a Sunday, in the very early morning on the ninth day of September 1951. I was the fourth child of my father Leonard and my mother Johanna. One of my first recollections is as a 3-year-old child. I was standing near a sunny wall at my home at Round Hill near Burnie, and someone holding a Box Brownie camera, said: 'Watch the birdie!' I kept looking and looking, but I did not see a birdie. I'll come back to this story later. The second memory is when I was older, around 7 years old, when I remember contemplating infinity, imagining space beyond space beyond space.

From the time I was 5, my family lived in a working-class housing estate in Burnie, called Acton Estate. It was the kind of neighbourhood where kids walked along the top railing of fences, played cricket in the road and ran everywhere they had to go. As a child I was physically healthy and most of my free time was spent at the beach, because I loved swimming. The people who were important to me were my mum, dad, grandmother Eva, brothers Kenny, Bobby and Allan, and my only sister Di. These people were important to me because they loved me, I loved them, and I knew I could trust them for basic things, like loyalty and protection.

Our home seemed large to my child's eyes, but I have been back to Grenville Street since as an adult and I have realized how small our housing commission home really was! I remember the unpretentious manner with which we related to one another; kids roaming relatively freely in bare feet and hand-me-down clothes, wrangling with and sticking up for one another, within a straight-talking yet mostly benevolent autocracy ruled over firmly by my father, and by my mother when dad was away working in the bush as an axeman. I have not regained that sense of carefree belonging and familiarity since those days at Grenville Street, where I knew that I belonged to my family and that my father, mother and grandmother were there to love, care for and protect me.

Other important influences in my childhood were my cat Tom, who rode patiently around in my pram and taught me about caring for someone beyond myself. The Hobbs kids next door, who enjoyed even less childhood luxuries than we Bugg kids, taught me about being happy with next to nothing of a material nature, and of speaking up for myself to win a share of whatever good things were on offer, such as freshly baked biscuits or who batted next in the backyard game of rounders. I was also influenced by the local Baptist church, of which I was a serious member. It was at Sunday School that I learned to 'do unto others as you would have them do unto you'. Other rules of living I learned around then were related to 'being a good girl'. I remember winning a competition at Sunday School for the person who could remain most silent for the longest time. I won it hands down, because I found it very simple to do as I was told.

I wanted to become a nurse so that I could 'evangelize' India. I had this arrogant notion that people in India needed Christianity and me, and I was filled with an altruistic zeal to save their souls, while I nursed their wounds. I imagined myself as an all-encompassing helper. By the time I decided to do nursing, I had lost these ideas and settled instead for the joys of the practice itself, plus the kudos of acquiring certificates and having a full-time, reliable job. My personal approach to practice was conscientious. I won the hospital medal for the 'best bedside manner', and even though I know I was worthy of that prize, I suspect that the award was really for being a very hard-working nurse. In the second year of my general training I stopped running around at full speed and with immense anxiety, and actually noticed that the people in the beds were humans, with all the hopes and fears I possessed.

There were many childhood ways of seeing the world that I brought with me into adulthood, but I'll focus on two I mentioned before – the memories of the little girl standing in front of the sunny wall and the infinity-imagining 7-year-old, who won the 'best child' award in Sunday School. The little girl waiting for the birdie is the optimistic adult in me now, who waits patiently for something lovely to happen. Sometimes I'm disappointed, and sometimes I'm thrilled by what transpires, but I retain a sense of anticipation and, to some extent, trust and patience. The little girl in Sunday School still knows how to stay quiet when it matters, and she works hard at doing things correctly and on time. She organizes herself well and puts a lot of time into pleasing other people, while imagining deep and mysterious concepts, often of a metaphysical nature.

Some 'rules for living' formed in my childhood have been transferred into my adult work life. I'm not in clinical practice now, but when I was, I always tried to treat people well, in the hope that they would treat me well in return. This rule did not always work, as the people I was 'doing unto' did not necessarily live by the same rule. This meant that I spent a lot of years in selfless service, giving so much of myself to patients, and not expecting anything back. After many years I became a reflective practitioner and, among many huge insights, I realized that I was so busy giving of myself that I did not leave enough space for people to give anything back to me. This came to a head one day when a woman in a postnatal ward gave me a hug for some simple words I offered her. I stayed still and silent and she was able to give me a hug. In my journaling later, I was able to see that my rule for living had been applied so conscientiously that it had kept me from receiving the very thing I hoped for most from my work – the love of the people for whom I cared. This insight was important for learning about myself and my relationships with other people, and it has been applied in many different ways in my life and work since that initial reflection.

Summary

In this section I suggested how you could recall and record your childhood memories in relation to who you are now as an adult and a clinician. I guided you through a reflective exercise, in which you responded to structured questions. This exercise was to demonstrate reflective questions and responses. I shared my own responses to this reflector, to show that simple yet meaningful connections can be made between early childhood memories of who we were as a child and who we have become as an adult and practitioner.

The role of a critical friend

Sometimes external perspectives can spark interest and involvement in reflection, and move personal responses to questions beyond your present field of vision. A critical friend can offer external perspectives to extend your reflective capacity. 'Critical' in this sense does not mean criticizing, but being prepared to ask important questions and make tentative suggestions to unseat previous perceptions, to find other possibilities and insights.

A critical friend is chosen by you as someone you trust and respect, to assist you with your reflection. In this way the relationship is akin to mentorship, although with time and trust a delegated clinical supervisor could also fill this role. Because it requires professional respect and confidentiality, a critical friendship is initiated ideally by the person requiring guidance, and not as a delegated responsibility to a relative stranger working in the organization.

The role of a critical friend is to listen and respond to your reflections about clinical incidents and to assist you in making some sense of them. A critical friend realizes that they are not meant to be the person with answers to every dilemma that you might raise; rather, the role is to encourage you to find the answers yourself. By a well-timed question or a spontaneous supportive comment, a critical friend provides the necessary support and stimulation for you to be the main 'sense-maker' of your reflections.

On the whole, reflective practice centres on the work of the reflecting clinician – that is, it does not make judgements about other people's practices. This means that reflective practice requires deep thought on an individual level and the danger of that is in not being able to see the practice constraints operating in the whole situation. A critical friend can help you see the 'wider picture' and broaden your possibilities for awareness and change.

Sharing practice stories requires courage, especially when less than best practice is revealed. It takes courage and a fair measure of maturity to admit that you are not invincible, that you make mistakes sometimes, or that you could have acted better in a situation. A critical friend hears what you have to say, and lets you talk it out as fully as you can, while being non-judgemental about you as a person.

Critical friends listen more than they talk, and they avoid making early foreclosures on what they think might be the issues at hand. A critical friend allows you to talk as much as you need to, in order to give a full description of the incident that occurred, so that there will be more substance to reflect on together. By encouraging you to talk, they will allow you to come to your own awareness. They may ask a question here or there to clarify what you have said, and to point out inconsistencies in your account if they become apparent.

One of the most important parts of a reflective story is its emotional content, because if you can identify your feelings you can begin to reflect on why they are as they are, and what you can learn from them. A critical friend can encourage you to express how you really felt about something that you have identified as problematic, and contained within that disclosure may be some clues as to the nature and the effects of the problem itself and how it relates to you and your practice.

Sometimes a critical friend jots down notes of what seem to be the salient points as you speak, rather than interrupt your flow of your ideas. The critical friend may also take special interest in the specific words you use, which suggest the emotional content of the story and the sense you have made of your experiences. If your story is very brief, or it lacks sufficient details on which to reflect, your critical friend may encourage you to elaborate further.

A critical friend is willing to help you in a supportive way, to challenge you to improve your reflective practice. To do this well, there must be a sense of trust, respect, rapport and enough time and space to allow you to come to your own awareness.

One of the ways in which you can be encouraged to go beyond your initial interpretation of your work issues is to explore the answers to questions which trigger reflection. Some reflective questions are suggested in the next section.

Encouraging reflective questioning

In Chapters 4, 5 and 6 of this book, relating to technical, practical and emancipatory reflection respectively, you will find lists of questions that you can pose about the procedural, interpersonal relationships and power aspects of your work. They are specific questions to guide you in uncovering insights into your work and to make you a happier and more effective clinician.

Some questions are not listed easily, because they come up as a conversation continues, but the chances are that they will emerge appropriately if your critical friend is attentive to the content and flow of what you are saying. Remember that not all questions have answers and some are worth asking for their rhetorical value. One of the benefits of asking questions in this process may be the realization that it is OK to leave discussions open-ended and that quick-fix solutions are not always necessary or appropriate.

Whereas the reflective questions that follow are not 'the definitive list', they may be useful cues for you or your prospective critical friend to get you started on cycles of deeper reflection.

The reflection begins with a practice story, which describes the 'who, when, what, where, why and how' of a particular clinical situation. If the person telling the story is having difficulty in maintaining the flow of the account, some prompts may be given, such as:

What happened then?
Who was involved?
What was your part in the situation?
How did that make you feel?

If there is a departure from the main theme of the conversation and it is time to refocus, prompts can be given, such as:

You were saying before . . .
Let's go back to where you were talking about . . .

The questions used thereafter depend entirely on the content and flow of the story and these are best exemplified in Kyah's practice story on p. 66.

Summary

This section described the role of a critical friend, to whom you give permission to ask questions of you and the practice issues on which you are reflecting. This external perspective can spark your interest and involvement in reflection, and move your personal responses to broader insights beyond your present perceptions. By being prepared to ask important questions and make tentative suggestions to unseat your previous perceptions, your critical friend helps you find other possibilities and insights.

The Taylor model of reflection

Given Schön's (1987) contention that successful reflection requires some coaching, this section provides an easy guide to successful reflection using a systematic flow approach. The 'Taylor model of reflection' uses a mnemonic device using the word REFLECT, to represent Readiness, Exercising thought, Following systematic processes, Leaving oneself open to answers, Enfolding insights, Changing awareness and Tenacity in maintaining reflection. This section begins with a diagrammatical representation of the model (see Figure 2.1), followed by a detailed explanation of each part of the flow.

Explanation of the diagrammatic representation

Diagrams of models always present a problem – of how to represent interrelated concepts in two-dimensional form and somehow achieve a sense of movement, flow and dynamism. Figure 2.1 attempts to demonstrate the systematic flow of reflection, in and through the world of healthcare practice, within the context of self in relation to other people, within the realities of internal historical, cultural, economic, social and political constraints, orbited by and in contact with external forces and influences. Immediately, you can appreciate the complex intentions of a relatively simple diagram, which cannot possibly fulfil these multilayered conceptual expectations. This is the difficulty of models of most kinds.

Author's reflection

When I was about 7, my eldest brother Ken had the task of creating a model of the solar system for a school project. I remember the awe I felt as he explained that the planets orbit the central sun, depicted most nobly by a large orange. I guess that this task is common to many classrooms across the world, and I had to recreate the solar system model when I arrived at senior levels of primary school. I could see from my shaky model of overhandled fruit and tenuous wire and string that our world depended on the orderly movement of our earth around the sun for our light and warmth, and that this rotation was fundamental to our survival.

When it came to describing infinity, however, there was no model to show the endlessness of space. Ken just moved his hands in an onward circular waving motion and said: 'Infinity is space beyond space beyond space – there is no end.' When I could not handle the mental gymnastics of this concept and tried to ask about the ultimate limits of space, he simply reiterated: 'There is no end; it just goes on forever.'

As far as I can remember, these examples were my first experiences of models and since that time I have seen the benefit of representing grand ideas with simple images.

Describing the model

The globe at the centre of the Figure 2.1 represents your world of practice, that is, all of the contextual features within and acting upon the setting in which you work. The REFLECT bands represent the systematic flow of reflective processes in and through the world of practice, preparing you for, and reacting to, the dynamic tension of your workplace.

Reflection as the REFLECT process is represented as a flow, rather than as steps, to show the ongoing and seamless connections between the reflective processes that permeate and flow in and through the human and material matrix of the sphere of practice. The flow of reflective processes may be rapid or slow, protracted or truncated, shallow or deep, bursting through the sphere of practice in unexpected places, in response to workplace circumstances, or being directed purposefully by you through the matrix of the world of practice, depending on the clinical issues within your work context and the internal and external constraints operating at any given time.

Reflective processes go within, through, around and across the sphere of practice, taking reflexive turns as they dive into and out of clinical issues and workplace phenomena. Your practice world is not neat and static, rather it is moving constantly, turning up, down and around, changing shape within itself due to its own internal context and constraints, and evolving, distorting and indenting, due to pressures and influences from the external constraints that constantly orbit, touch and sometimes collide with the sphere of practice. The diagram represents the external constraints by the structures which look like orbiting electrons.

External constraints, pressures and influences are historical, cultural, economic, social, political and personal forces and have a bearing on your

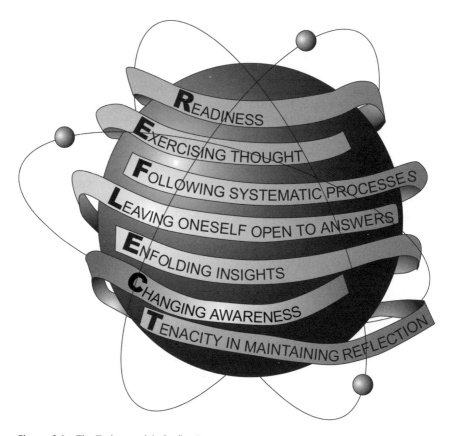

Figure 2.1 The Taylor model of reflection

workplace and practices. These constraints include pressures and influences, such as environmental factors, politics, consumer and professional communities, health patterns and initiatives, from general and global levels to specific and focused national, regional and local levels. All of the external constraints are complex and interrelated, always present, sometimes unpredictably, in an unstable and often chaotic external environment. For example, healthcare agencies comply with national, regional and local demands and expectations for accreditation, and money to provide essential services is allocated to a healthcare system competing for limited funds for maintaining and expanding its local healthcare services. Thus, the world of healthcare practice is 'under attack' constantly from internal and external constraints, while attempting to create stable, healing environments and services for clients, whose health needs increase exponentially, as the mean age of the population increases.

The internal context of your practice world is made up of the complex and relatively unpredictable matrix of human and material entities, as people relate to self and to other people, within the determinants of internal historical, cultural, economic, social, political and personal constraints. People and constraints are fundamental to healthcare organizations, because the nature of healthcare systems is that people must interact in complex roles and relationships, and they must operate within limits and boundaries placed on and within the healthcare culture. The constraints of historical norms, cultural expectations and competition for money, power and personal authority act as obstructions, retardants and challenges to practice that are negotiated by reflective processes as they flow in, around or through your practice world, depending on the degree of opposition. Interpersonal communication and contestation is difficult and challenging in most contexts and healthcare settings are no exception.

The seamless flow of reflective processes include Readiness, Exercising thought, Following systematic processes, Leaving oneself open to answers, Enfolding insights, Changing awareness and Tenacity in maintaining reflection. These processes are the proactive, interactive and reactive means by which the sources and effects of the unpredictable and inevitable obstructions, attacks and challenges in your workplace are identified and worked through to restore, maintain and possibly improve the overall integrity of the world of practice. Due to the ongoing severity of the challenges on and in your practice, other means are also necessary to bolster the integrity of the workplace, so these reflective processes do not claim to be the panacea for all the ills and challenges of practice. Rather, the reflective processes depicted as REFLECT provide one of many ways through which the sphere of practice can be restored, maintained and improved. Given the enormity of the task of being a practitioner, and the unpredictability of the context in which you work, you are well advised to engage actively in reflective processes, such as those offered in this model depicted by the mnemonic device REFLECT.

Reflector

What is your sphere of practice like? What pressures and constraints are within your practice world? What external pressures and constraints act on that world? Do you imagine that reflection in and on your practice will assist you? If not, why not? If yes, how?

Readiness

As the first requirement, you need to take the time and space to be ready to reflect. Given the busy nature of work settings, it is not always possible to take much time or to even find a space for reflection, but it can be done very simply.

Readiness to reflect comes from silence from within oneself, even if it is only for a moment. All it takes is for you to 'go inside' yourself to that quiet space within. Being ready by being silent, even for a microsecond, prepares you to centre from an inner place of quietness, and from there to move outwards through thought to action. Being ready to reflect through momentary silence assumes an orientation towards reflective processes and sets your intention, because your inner readiness acknowledges that reflective practices are effective, and are valuable enough to spend some time in engaging actively with them on and in your practice world.

Readiness for reflection also comes from some knowledge of concepts and a willingness to practise skills shown already by other reflective practitioners to be useful. The accumulation of some knowledge and skills in readiness for reflection is akin to starting out on a journey with some idea of the itinerary and knowing in general how to get where you are going, but not necessarily with a detailed knowledge of the landscape, or even a sense of the eventualities along the way.

Getting ready to reflect and to maintain a reflective attitude to your life and work requires the qualities of taking and making time, making the effort, being determined, having courage and knowing how to use humour. These qualities are discussed in this chapter, and they will serve you well as you develop reflective knowledge and skills. Even if your levels of these qualities are low and almost imperceptible, they can be nurtured and strengthened through ongoing reflective practice.

Practice story

Kyah is a 23-year-old physiotherapist, who has been working in an acute healthcare setting for one year. Her clinical experience has been mainly in orthopaedics, working with a wide range of clients, suffering from conditions as diverse as sports injuries and degenerative bone diseases. As part of her clinical supervision process, Kyah's recently appointed mentor, Kate, suggested that they use Taylor's REFLECT model to work together through issues in Kyah's work.

At first, Kyah was resistant to the idea, arguing with Kate that, in her practice, physiotherapy focuses on complex biotechnical aspects of the musculoskeletal system and mobility, and that her undergraduate degree and subsequent clinical experience had prepared her for any issues that might arise in her work. In response, Kate reminded Kyah of a recent problem they had been discussing, in which a client had complained about Kyah's 'attitude', alluding to something unrelated to her technical proficiency as a physiotherapist. Kate explained that she would take the role of a critical friend and guide Kyah through the reflective process.

With some initial reluctance, but being perplexed about what the client meant by her 'attitude', Kyah agreed to undertake the reflective process within scheduled clinical supervision sessions.

Kate encouraged Kyah to recount a recent clinical situation, in which she had been attending to the postoperative physiotherapy needs of a 50-year-old recreational golfer, George, who required a right shoulder reconstruction. Although the postoperative period was uneventful in terms of the technical aspects of care, Kyah noticed that George was often emotionally irritable in her presence, even though he complied with her postoperative directions for his shoulder care. The situation intensified when Kyah asked George's partner Harold to leave the bedside, so she could attend to George's physio. Shortly after George's discharge, the head of department received a written complaint from George indicating that he was offended by Kyah's attitude towards him.

Critical friend response

Kyah: *So, what happens now? Where do we start?*
Kate: *We start by getting ready to reflect. There are a number of things you can do Kyah, but the best way to begin is by being silent and centred.*
Kyah: *What do you mean by being centred?*
Kate: *It's a way of going within yourself, to find a quiet place, away from your mind chatter and busyness. You start from a clear, empty space. Quietness is the key, even if it is just for a few moments. Sit comfortably, breathe quietly for a minute or so and empty your head.*

Exercising thought

Reflection is mediated through thinking on and in experiences in your personal and work life. Turning on to and tuning into thought is essential for reflective practice, because healthcare practitioners are thinking professionals who use their knowledge, skills and humanity in purposeful care. Reflection is the 'throwing back of thoughts and memories, in cognitive acts such as thinking, contemplation, meditation and any other form of attentive consideration, in order to make sense of them, and to make contextually appropriate changes if they are required' (Taylor 2000: 3). Reflection assumes that thoughts are energized into action. For example, tacit knowledge, or knowing in action, the kind of sophisticated knowledge of which clinicians may not be entirely aware, can be made explicit through exercising thought in reflection during or after practice (Schön 1987).

There are many strategies that can be used when exercising thought in systematic reflection. Some inspire reflection, others guide, and some inspire and guide simultaneously. A kitbag of strategies are described in this chapter, which can be used and adapted in any combination and quantity to suit the situation.

When you are exercising thought in reflection, remember to be spontaneous, express yourself freely, remain open to ideas, choose a time and place to suit you, be prepared personally, and choose suitable reflective methods.

Practice story

After a short silence, Kyah's practice story continued. She explained to Kate that up until this time, she had relied on her practice knowledge, skills and problem-solving abilities to approach clinical difficulties. She had not really given much thought to using systematic reflective processes regularly, even though she was committed to improving her practice and learning from her clinical experiences. She practised physiotherapy thoughtfully, but she realized her thinking had been mostly in relation to the technical aspects of care, and that she had a tendency to focus solely on the client's affected body part when attending to care. She asked Kate about the kind of thinking necessary for successful reflection.

Critical friend response

Kate: *When you think in a work situation, what do you do?*
Kyah: *I'm not sure I know what you mean.*
Kate: *Imagine you're watching yourself think. What are you doing?*
Kyah: *Well, I guess I do what I've been taught. My thinking is pretty much regulated and focused on the affected body part. Most of the time, I think according to a clinical problem-solving approach I've been taught, but it doesn't always mean the outcomes are one hundred per cent successful in all cases.*
Kate: *Do you always stay totally focused in your thinking on the clinical problem?*
Kyah: *No, not always, sometimes my thoughts wander a bit, or they become a bit chaotic, especially if I have a huge workload and there's a lot on my mind.*

Kate: *As a physiotherapist, you've been taught how to think clinic-*
ally, and to focus on the care of a body part, but there may
be times when this does not always help in the totality of the
situation. When we exercise thought intentionally in reflec-
tion, we direct our attention towards the full clinical context
and make our thinking purposeful.

Following systematic processes

When concepts and ideas are complex it is useful to break them down into smaller parts to make them more manageable. Reflection has the potential to be very complex, especially when practice issues and problems are in focus. For this reason, the Taylor model imagines three types of reflection – technical, practical and emancipatory, based on ways of knowing and Habermas' 'knowledge-constitutive interests', described in Chapter 3.

Technical reflection helps you to improve your instrumental action through technical control and manipulation in devising and improving procedural approaches to your work. Practical reflection helps you to understand the interpersonal basis of human experiences and offers you the potential for creating knowledge, by interpreting the meaning of lived experience, context and subjectivity, and the potential for change, based on raised awareness of the nature of a wide range of communicative matters pertaining to healthcare practice. Emancipatory reflection leads to 'transformative action', which seeks to free you from taken-for-granted assumptions and oppressive forces, which limit you and your practice, by critiquing the power relationships in your workplace and offering you raised awareness and a new sense of informed consciousness to bring about positive social and political change. No type of reflection is better than another; each has its own value for different purposes, and each type can be used alone or in combination with the other types.

Systematic questioning is the basis of all the reflective processes. For example, technical reflection encourages scientific reasoning, using questions within the steps of assessing and planning, implementing and evaluating. In 'assessing and planning' you set up the premises for rational thinking by making an initial assessment of the problem and planning for the development of an argument. 'Implementing' is the part of the technical reflection process in which you develop an argument by analysing the issues and assumptions operating in the situation. In 'evaluating' you review the problem in the light of all the information gained through the process of technical reflection. The outcomes of technical reflection can be immediate, if the process has been shared with, and the findings endorsed by, the key people who are in a position to influence and ratify healthcare practice. Technical reflection has the potential for allowing you to think critically and to reason scientifically, so that you can critique and adapt procedures and policies. You may also be able to predict likely outcomes for similar procedures and improve many work practices through objective and systematic lines of enquiry.

Through systematic questioning processes in practical reflection you will be assisted to understand the interpersonal basis of human experiences and the potential for creating new knowledge, in your lived experience, context and subjectivity. Practical reflection is a process of experiencing, interpreting and learning. Experiencing involves retelling a practice story so that you experience it again in as much detail as possible. Interpreting involves clarifying and explaining the meaning of a communicative action situation. Learning involves creating new insights and integrating them into your existing awareness and knowledge. Change is possible in practical reflection through new insights from raised awareness.

The systematic processes of emancipatory reflection will assist you to analyse critically personal, political, sociocultural, historical or economic contextual features, and constraints that may have a bearing on your practice. Emancipatory reflection provides you with a means of critiquing the status quo in the workplace and offers you a new sense of informed consciousness to bring about positive change. The process of emancipatory reflection for change is *praxis*, which offers you the means for change through collaborative processes that analyse and challenge existing forces and distortions brought about by the dominating effects of power in human interaction. Emancipatory reflection provides a process to construct, confront, deconstruct and reconstruct your practice. Construction of practice incidents allows you to describe, in words and other creative images and representations, a work scene played out previously, bringing to mind all of the aspects and constraints of the situation.

Deconstruction involves asking analytical questions regarding the situation, which are aimed at locating and critiquing all the aspects of that situation. Confrontation occurs when you focus on your part in the scenario with the intention of seeing and describing it as clearly as possible. Reconstruction puts the scenario together again with transformative strategies for managing change in the light of the new insights.

All kinds of knowledge can be generated through reflection, and healthcare professionals can benefit from a range of reflective processes. The first set of questions you should ask yourself in choosing a specific type or combination of types of reflection consists of: 'What do I want to know through reflection?' 'Why do I want to know it?' 'What questions will stimulate and guide my reflections and lead me to the answers I am seeking?' 'Is my primary focus on work procedures, human interaction or power relationships, or a combination of these interests?'

Finding a balance for using types of knowledge and reflection is important, because knowledge exists for all sorts of purposes and the reflective techniques healthcare professionals use will depend on what they need to achieve. The division of reflection into technical, practical and emancipatory is artificial and contrived for convenience – each type does not exist in isolation from another and they are not mutually exclusive. If you can develop a reflective consciousness based on balance and context, it will serve you well in deciding how to reflect on any issues which present themselves in your practice.

Practice story

From the description thus far, Kate suggested that as Kyah's practice issue was not a technical one and did not appear to be about explicit politics, practical reflection (see Chapter 5) would be the best approach for experiencing, interpreting and learning from her interpersonal issue with George. With Kate's guidance, Kyah responded to the questions within the process.

I was working in the ortho postop unit and I was very busy, with three clients back from surgery that day and six others, including George, who were well into their postop rehab. I saw George around 3 p.m. and I still had to see four other clients before 5 p.m. George's friend Harold was visiting and they were having a coffee together and an intense conversation about something. The coffee smelt fantastic and I was keen to get on with my work and go for a coffee break myself. I asked Harold to leave us for 10 minutes or so, and even though he didn't say so as such, I could see that George was very annoyed with me. I don't know why. I was there to do my work and even though I was aware something was wrong, I felt peeved. I had work to do, and I needed to do it.

Critical friend response

As Kyah recounted the story, her voice quickened and became shrill and louder.

Kyah: *Listen to me. I'm sounding defensive about this.*

Kate: *Let's look closely at the interaction. What were your hopes for that interaction with George?*

Kyah: *I wanted to do his physio, so he could go home within a day or so, as he had hoped.*

Kate: *How were your hopes for George related to your ideals of good physiotherapy practice?*

Kyah:	*Good physiotherapy helps clients regain musculoskeletal function to an optimal level and that was happening.*
Kate:	*So what else was happening? You said before that you asked Harold to leave so you could attend to the physio. Let's go back to that.*
Kyah:	*Well, I went in, walked past Harold, looked straight at George, and asked Harold to leave.*
Kate:	*In what tone of voice?*
Kyah:	*The usual tone of voice I have for work is quicker and higher – I guess it has a ring of importance. I talk differently at work. Work is not like being at home, where I can afford to be more at ease. I have a ton of things to do at work and I need clients' cooperation to get them done properly and on time. I guess I'm detached and professional at work.*
Kate:	*What are the sources in your life for your way of communicating in a detached, professional way at work?*
Kyah:	*I grew up in a medical family – mum and dad are both doctors and I have a sister who's a doctor and a brother who's a social worker. My training impressed the need for me to stay detached clinically, so the main focus is on the client's problems. There was some mention of holistic approaches, but the focus was really on diagnosing and treating affected body parts.*

Leaving oneself open to answers

Reflective processes do not necessarily provide you with indisputable 'truth' or correct answers to apply universally to all clinical situations, issues and problems. Even so, reflection may bring insights and partial 'truths' that may have some relevance for your practice. However, the first insight may not always be the best or the only flash of awareness that can enhance your work, so remain open to ideas so that they have a chance to grow, change or even disappear. Jumping to early conclusions may inhibit further insights and solutions, so be prepared for twists and turns in your thinking.

Some questions may remain puzzles to which you will always be seeking some insights, and that is OK, because sometimes what you learn in the search is more beneficial than what you find in the discovery. Enjoy the openness in reflective practice and realize that your answers will not be absolutes, but consider them as tentative answers to problems and issues that may need revisiting later. Be prepared to live with uncertainty and let go of your need to know indisputably. A sense of openness and preparedness for what comes puts you in a state of readiness to entertain multiple possible answers to issues and problems encountered in rapidly changing clinical contexts.

Practice story

Kate and Kyah continued their discussion about Kyah's interaction with George. Kate assisted Kyah to learn from her practice story, by asking some questions to prompt reflection.

Critical friend response

Kate: *Kyah, what does this story about George, Harold and you tell you about your expectations of yourself?*

Kyah: *I expect myself to act and communicate professionally at all times at work.*

Kate: *And that means?*

Kyah: *I keep myself to myself, I focus on a client's issue, and I speak in a professional and focused way, to get the work done.*

Kate: *Does that always work the best in every case?*

Kyah: *Well, I suppose it doesn't, does it? Something about that inter-action with George went sour, even though I followed my usual way of interacting. It wasn't the homosexual thing, that's no big deal for me, I can assure you. Maybe something was going on between George and Harold that I walked into – they were in an intense one to one. I was polite, but maybe I was 'plastic' polite – not real and genuine, just following a prescription for playing it tightly and getting on with my work. It might have been something altogether different from what I'm thinking. I'm not sure. I'll need some time to think about it.*

Enfolding insights

As you remain open to ideas, enfold insights from multiple sources and mix new insights into present understandings. You may decide to use a variety of reflective processes and strategies as an individual or within a group and you may enlist critical friendships to assist in enfolding insights.

A critical friend can offer external perspectives to extend your reflective capacity, by asking important questions and making tentative suggestions to unseat your previous perceptions, to find other possibilities and insights.

A critical friend realizes that they are not meant to be the person with answers to every dilemma that you might raise. The role is to encourage you to find the answers yourself. A critical friend hears what you have to say, and lets you talk it out as fully as you can.

Enfold insights and let them rest a while. What arises out of the insights will be all the richer if you allow them to gather, coalesce and merge into deeper and more meaningful possibilities for your life and practice.

> ### Practice story
>
> *Kate and Kyah met a fortnight later, during which time Kyah had time to think over their previous conversation and enfold other insights into her practice story of caring for George.*

> ### Critical friend response
>
> Kyah: *This reflective practice process sure makes you think, doesn't it!*
> Kate: *Yes, so tell me what's been happening for you Kyah.*
> Kyah: *I've been thinking a lot about how I was in that interaction.*
> Kate: *Not about the what, but the . . .*
> Kyah: *. . . how! Yes, what I did was what I would usually do – focus on the client, get to the work in hand – 'Miss Efficiency' as usual. You keep referring to the interaction as between George, Harold and myself. I refer to it as between George and me. There was a third person in the interaction. Harold was there, talking intently with George and having a coffee, but I ignored him completely. It's like he was invisible, really. I didn't acknowledge Harold at all. I had my back to him and I didn't even look at him when I asked him to leave us. There was no real urgency in doing the physio then and there – it could have waited, really. George was due to go home within days, so most of the healing was happening. I'm beginning to think that 'one size does not fit all', when it comes to communicating at work!*

Changing awareness

Insights raise awareness and raised awareness in turn raises the possibility of change. Sometimes change is small, at local levels, and sometimes it is large, within wider contexts – it does not matter, as change is change and it shifts the status quo, if only in fractional amounts. Make small, manageable changes in preference to no changes at all.

Changing awareness through reflective practice often comes through examining the emotional content of your practice stories, because if you can identify your feelings, you can begin to reflect on why they are as they are, and what you can learn from them. Express how you really felt about something that you have identified as problematic, and contained within that disclosure may be some clues as to the nature and the effects of the problem itself and how it relates to you and your practice.

Practice story

Kyah shared her insights into herself and her practice of communicating at work. As her critical friend, Kate mostly listened quietly, keeping comfortable eye contact with Kyah and nodding her head. Kyah came to her own insights and Kate was to be there to listen, respond empathetically, and ask a question here and there.

Critical friend response

Kate: *So Kyah, will your story about George and Harold change the way you communicate at work?*

Kyah: *Definitely! It'll take a while to change my established patterns, but I'm going to try to slow down and take a wider scan of the situation when I'm with clients. I need to be aware of the client and anyone with them, instead of rush, rush – 'I'm very important, please do as I ask, now! 'I'm trying to tune into my tone of voice also. I've realized in the last week or so that I have a 'packaged niceness' approach, which includes me speaking in falsetto. I'm working on bringing my voice down a few octaves to a pitch I use in everyday conversations. I've realized the falsetto is about keeping my distance so I can get things done. It's like: 'Please return your tray tables to the normal position ready for landing' – my words and pitch direct clients, they don't really involve them in choices or relate to them on a one-to-one, genuine level. I guess it takes practice to be really at ease and in the moment with clients, especially on busy days!*

Tenacity in maintaining reflection

Demonstrate tenacity in your resolve to maintain reflection, so that you become a reflective practitioner for life. Some ways of maintaining reflective practice are by affirming yourself as a reflective practitioner, responding to the critiques, creating a daily habit, seeing things freshly, staying alert to practice, finding support systems, sharing reflection, getting involved in research and embodying reflective practice. These ideas are discussed in the last chapter of this book.

Affirm your worth as a reflective practitioner, by acknowledging your insights and how far you have come from who and how you were when you began, to who and how you are now. To be assured of the worth of reflection, you may need to respond to the critics, so that your investment in maintaining reflection does not suffer. To affirm your experience of reflection, it will be important to maintain the everydayness of your reflective practice, by using opportunities to take time out from the busyness of life to spend time in silence. Adopting a new way of seeing the events of everyday life can assist in maintaining reflective practice, by trying actively to keep a fresh perspective on ordinary aspects of life that you would otherwise have taken for granted. You can affirm your status as a reflective practitioner by staying alert to your practice, noticing the details that can keep you entrenched in unexamined clinical procedures, patterns of human relating and power-plays. Ascertain whether there are other clinicians engaged in reflective practice to encourage one another to maintain reflection. Share reflective experiences in your ward, department, private practice or organization, by organizing a professional development seminar or conference. There is wide scope for research incorporating reflective processes or centred on experiences of reflective practice. You will find advice on doing research, writing professional articles and presenting your work at conferences in Chapter 8 of this book. As a daily routine of life, begin to embody reflective practice, so that it becomes an integral part of who and how you are.

Reflector

Think of a change in lifestyle you promised yourself. It might be a New Year resolution, or an attempt to lose weight or give up smoking. What caused you to feel the need for a change? What plans did you make and put into action to bring about the change? In what ways were you successful/unsuccessful? Are any of these insights useful now to put into action to help you maintain a reflective approach to your life and work?

Summary

In this chapter I suggested that reflective practitioners need to nurture the qualities of taking and making time, making the effort, being determined, having courage and knowing how to use humour. A kitbag of strategies for reflecting was described, including writing, audiotaping, creating music, dancing, drawing, montage, painting, poetry, pottery, quilting, singing and videotaping, used in any combination you prefer. When you reflect I encouraged you to remember to be spontaneous, express yourself freely, remain open to ideas, choose a time and place to suit you, be prepared personally and choose suitable reflective methods. The role of a critical friend was described as a trusted and respected colleague, who assists you in reaching deeper levels of reflection by asking questions and encouraging you to challenge some of your assumptions and intentions. Reflective practice can take you to deeper levels of knowledge about yourself and your practice and the introductory ideas in this chapter can get you started. Lastly, this chapter provided you with the Taylor model of reflection, depicted by the mnemonic device REFLECT. This book elaborates on every aspect of the Taylor model, to give you confidence in being a reflective healthcare practitioner.

Key points

- It takes time, effort, determination, courage and humour to initiate and maintain effective reflection.
- There are many strategies you can use when engaging in systematic reflection.
- When you are reflecting, remember to be spontaneous, express yourself freely, remain open to ideas, choose a time and place to suit you, be prepared personally and choose suitable reflective methods.
- A good exercise to get you started on reflecting is to recall and record your childhood memories in relation to who you are now as an adult and a clinician, to discover some of the values and rules for living that influence your practice.
- A critical friend can offer external perspectives to extend your reflective capacity, by asking important questions and making tentative suggestions to unseat your previous perceptions, to find other possibilities and insights.
- One of the most important parts of a reflective story is its emotional content, because if you can identify your feelings, you can begin to reflect on why they are as they are, and what you can learn from them.

- One of the ways in which you can be encouraged to go beyond your initial interpretation of your work issues is to explore the answers to questions, which trigger reflection.
- As an easy guide, in a systematic flow approach to successful reflection, the 'Taylor model of reflection' uses a mnemonic device, REFLECT, to represent Readiness, Exercising thought, Following systematic processes, Leaving oneself open to answers, Enfolding insights, Changing awareness and Tenacity in maintaining reflection.

3 Types of reflection and being human in healthcare

Introduction

This chapter sounds a note of caution about the use of categories, before introducing three types of reflection you can use in your work, and adapt to your personal life if you wish. Empirical, interpretive and critical knowledge are connected to Habermas' 'knowledge-constitutive interests' to create technical, practical and emancipatory reflection. The relative merits and shortcomings of the types of reflection are described, to assist you in choosing the types to use for your practice. Lastly, I describe a model for being human in healthcare encounters, which can be combined with reflective processes to enhance your knowledge, skills and humanity in your practice.

Caution about categories

When concepts and ideas are complex it is useful to break them down into subsections to make them more manageable. Reflection has the potential to be very complex, especially when practice issues and problems are in focus. I describe three types of reflection, based on ways of knowing and Habermas' 'knowledge-constitutive interests', and emphasize they can be used in combination, because practice issues are often unpredictable and complex.

The complexity of knowledge has been recognized by postmodern thinkers (Baudrillard 1988; Giroux 1990; Rosenau 1992), who warn against accepting 'grand narratives' to explain human behaviour and natural phenomena. In other words, postmodernists argue that 'big' theories and categories of knowledge do not necessarily represent what we can rely on as 'truth'. Even so, in the absence of experience and prior knowledge, we need to start somewhere from a point of reference when things are relatively new and strange for us. While it is all very well for postmodernists to critique all-encompassing explanations of human life as being too generalized to matter on a personal level, sometimes we need guideposts and markers to channel our thinking.

In this chapter, I suggest that empirical knowledge comes from technical reflection, interpretive knowledge comes from practical reflection, and critical knowledge comes from emancipatory reflection. These categories have been written about previously in relation to education (Mezirow 1981) and research (Carr and Kemmis 1984). That these categories have been used successfully elsewhere suggests that they are useful, even though caution is needed in trying to fit ideas into categories.

It is important to consider these categories as ways of creating a temporary framework on which to hang certain broad principles. The tendency to create a structure fits the assumption that there are major paradigms, or worldviews of knowledge, which can account for particular ways of thinking. It would be shortsighted to have an absolute conviction that there are only three forms of knowledge and reflection. I do not intend to give that message to you. The categories I am suggesting here are ways of structuring your thinking until you have the confidence you need to disregard the conceptual boxes, so that you can roam freely in open fields of uncategorized knowledge and reflection.

The three forms of knowledge and reflection described in this chapter are complementary to one another, because they share common features and at times merge into one another. All three approaches use similar ways of thinking, even though in some cases it seems a fairly 'clean cut' decision as to the specific type of thinking to use in particular instances. For example, the tasks involved in technical reflection are best served by a high degree of rationality of a 'scientific model' kind. Even so, emancipatory reflection might include some aspects of scientific rationality – say, for example, if part of the process involves changing outmoded clinical procedures to those that can be shown to demonstrate better practice. Therefore, even though I differentiate three forms of reflection connected to three knowledge types, feel free to mix and match them according to your own needs, based on the assumption that all knowledge is integrated and everything that adds something to a solution or insight is equally important. In the future, when you become more adept at being a reflective practitioner, you may choose to reflect using a specific type, or to take a 'mixed bag' approach, because you will have gained expertise in knowing how to reflect according to the demands of a particular situation.

Empirical knowledge

Empirical knowledge is generated and tested through 'the scientific method': a set of rules for gaining knowledge through a systematic and rigorous procedure. Scientific inquiry ensures that knowledge can be tested over and over again and found to be accurate and consistent (reliability). It also ensures that it tests what it actually intends (validity), rather than other factors that are extra or unnoticed (extraneous variables). To achieve this, scientific knowledge is rendered as free as possible from the distorting influences of people, such as their prejudices, intentions and emotions (subjectivity). In other words, empirical knowledge needs to show that due consideration has been given to achieving objectivity.

Another requirement of empirical knowledge is that the only research questions that can be asked legitimately are those which can be structured in ways that can be observed and analysed (by empirico-analytical means) and measured by numbers, percentages and statistics (quantified). This is why research using the scientific method is also referred to as empirico-analytical and/or quantitative research. The scientific method reduces areas of inquiry to their smallest parts (reductionism) in order to study them. This idea assumes that all empirical knowledge is waiting to be discovered and assembled, as absolute knowledge. The reason empirical knowledge is reductionist is that it reduces areas of interest to their smallest parts. It also attempts to find cause and effect links between certain objects and subjects (variables), which are controlled and manipulated carefully. Empirical knowledge confirms or disputes the degree of certainty in cause and effect relationships, by demonstrating significance statistically. This allows empirical knowledge to claim to be predictive and generalizable with some confidence that the conclusions are truthful, real and trustworthy, and not happening by chance. The outcomes are achieved mainly through rational deductive thinking processes, which move systematically from broad to focused inferences.

In summary, the scientific method generates and validates empirical knowledge through rigorous means such as reliability, validity, and control and manipulation of variables, to produce objective data that can be quantified to demonstrate the degree of statistical significance in cause and effect relationships. The outcomes of this method for the generation of empirical knowledge include description of what is, prediction for what might be, and change through new knowledge discoveries. The success of empirical knowledge is evident in healthcare through the constant evolution of newer and safer technical procedures.

Reflector

Think of two examples of work procedures that represent empirical knowledge. How can you be sure that you can 'trust' these procedures to be safe and effective? It might help you to judge each procedure against the criteria for empirical knowledge described in this section.

Interpretive knowledge

People are the focus of interpretive knowledge, because this form of knowledge features their perceptions of their life experiences and their ability to communicate them. The underlying concepts of interpretive knowledge include interpersonal understanding through attention to lived experience, context and subjectivity.

Lived experience means knowing, through living a life in a particular time, place and set of circumstances. Humans have the potential for reflecting on lived experiences. Other living beings such as animals may also have lived experiences, but they are unable to communicate them through spoken language and reflection. Therefore, lived experience in this sense is described in terms of human existence only.

Dreyfus (1979 in Benner and Wrubel 1989: 83) claims that 'we are able to move around in the everyday world because our understanding is always situated and our actions are typically only as orderly as the situation demands'. Novel situations may be managed with reference to like situations of which people have had previous experience. This seems true of healthcare practice. Practitioners are very familiar with the work setting and circumstances, and thus they feel ready for what may transpire as part of the working day. Healthcare professionals have a knack of knowing what to do and how to do it in certain unforeseen circumstances. One explanation for this is the interpretive knowledge they have developed through their lived experience of being a practitioner.

Reflector

What is your lived experience of your healthcare profession in relation to the ways in which you practise your work? It might help to think about the values that guide your practice and determine the way you relate to people in your workplace. Do you 'walk your talk' about how to be an effective healthcare professional? For example, if you think that honesty is a necessary value for practice, are you always honest in every situation? If your lived experience of your practice does not fit with your espoused values, how does that make you feel?

Context means all of the features of the time and place in which people find themselves, in which their lives are located and their realities are embodied. People live their daily lives in the moment, yet they also remain connected to their past and future (Heidegger 1962). People cannot help but be placed, and involved in, a particular time and place, which gives a sense of familiarity. Context provides relative stability for daily activity, because so many things can happen in an ever-changing world. Healthcare professionals work out what to do and how to do it in any situation by making personal applications to their own life issues, worries and stories, and to their sense of time, habits and favoured rituals and patterns of behaviour in various groups. They also pay attention to how they feel and what sense they make of it based on experience.

Subjectivity refers to the individual's sensing of inner and external events, which is appropriate for themselves. Subjectivity includes personal experiences and 'truths' that may or may not be like other people's subjective experiences and 'truths'. *Intersubjectivity* refers to how individuals take account of one another in the social world to make sense of their experiences. Healthcare occurs in social contexts in which intersubjective meanings are generated, because clinicians interpret their work experiences from their respective person-to-person viewpoints.

In summary, interpretive knowledge emerges from the perspectives of people engaged personally in their lives and it includes and values what people feel and think. Judgements as to the usefulness and 'truthfulness' of people's accounts are based on relative indicators, such as the nature of lived experience, context and subjectivity.

Critical knowledge

Critical knowledge is derived from some key ideas in critical social science, which emerged after World War I. A group of philosophers of the Frankfurt School decided that a way of generating knowledge other than through the scientific method was needed to open up new thinking about human knowing and experience, in order to prevent future wars and domination by oppressive regimes. Critical knowledge has the potential to be emancipatory – that is, it can free people from the oppression of their entrenched social and personal conditions.

The need for emancipation comes from the assumption that certain people, in the circumstances in which they find themselves, may suffer oppression and constraints of some kind, by other people and regimes. Freedom from oppression comes from being aware that it is happening in terms of historical, social, political, cultural and economic determinants and from finding the means to do something about it. Critical knowledge and theorizing seek to look into what is promoted as the status quo of various repressive social contexts, to discover and expose the forces that maintain them for their particular advantages. This means that critical theorists look at the way life is and ask how it might be different and better for the majority of people, not just for the privileged few.

Critical knowledge includes consideration of lived experience, context and intersubjectivity; other related key ideas are false consciousness, hegemony, reification, emancipation and empowerment. You will see that the first three words describe the oppressive potential of social life, and the last two provide some optimism about how repressive circumstances can be overcome.

False consciousness is the 'systematic ignorance that the members of . . . society have about themselves and their society' (Fay 1987: 27). Critical knowledge attempts to critique firmly held individual and collective ignorance to change this self-defeating consciousness and transform society itself. For example, the women's movement of the twentieth century finally identified and challenged women's oppression by men after centuries of assimilating male dominance. One of the reasons western women remained oppressed for so long was the firmly held ignorance of the oppression itself, perpetuated by the unquestioned acceptance of male-dominated cultural practices. Healthcare professionals might relate to the concept of false consciousness as clinicians working in bureaucratic settings where oppressive daily rituals remain unquestioned, because they are unnoticed. For example, some professionals may continue to accept power structures in their workplace, such as interpersonal relationships that keep them subservient to other professionals in authority positions, because in trying to maintain their employment they do not even think to 'rock the boat' and critique and challenge oppressive forces. The difficulty with false consciousness is the systematic ignorance itself, because it is sustained by unawareness, so it takes deep and sustained reflection to even uncover some issues as problematic.

Hegemony means the ascendancy or domination of one power over another. In a critical social science interpretation, it refers to the ways in which some social systems, and the people in them, give the impression that they are unassailable, and that the conditions they have produced are not only good, but also appropriate for the people over whom they have control. In healthcare, this might mean that some professionals come to think that the hospital bureaucracy is not only necessary but also conducive to their welfare, and that the oppressive elements within it, such as dominating relationships and difficult work conditions, cannot and should not be changed. Thus, hegemony would have some healthcare professionals believe that they can do little to change their work lives. Hegemonic influences maintain the status quo and are resistant to change, so clinicians need to critique taken-for-granted assumptions about everyday practices, in order to identify and change them in their workplace.

Reflector

Can you identify hegemonic practices where you work? What are they? Why are they so powerful? What, if anything, can be done about them? If your responses to this reflector are pessimistic of change at this point, take heart, as emancipatory reflection, as described in this book, may provide some optimistic options for action.

Fay (1987: 92) explains that *reification* means 'making into a thing'. He defines it as 'taking what are essential activities and treating them as if they operated according to a given set of laws independently of the wishes of the social actors who engage in them'. These laws of social life are assigned a power of their own. For example, a female healthcare professional may assume that, as a woman, it is a given that she will be subordinate to males in other better paid roles, so she acts in accordance with that assumption and fetches, carries, cleans up and generally accedes to the male professionals' directions. Reified practices are rich sources of reflection and they can be identified and changed through systematic questioning and action.

Emancipation means freedom, and it infers that one is free from something and free towards something. Critical knowledge claims to be helpful in emancipating people to be liberated from their present oppressive conditions towards empowering conditions. Emancipation for healthcare professionals, therefore, can mean that they experience freedom from the limitations of their own and other people's expectations and roles, to be free to adopt expansive self-aware and socially aware practices.

Empowerment is the process of giving and accepting power. Critical knowledge is geared towards helping people to find their own power, to liberate them from their oppressive circumstances and self-understandings in those circumstances. Empowerment for healthcare professionals may come about when they have used reflection to work through a radical critique of their personal and professional roles and conditions and have liberated themselves to other possibilities. In a practical sense this may be something seemingly simple, such as being the patients' advocate, or demonstrating and asserting their worth as professionals in the health team. While these examples may not seem extraordinary, they can amount to major changes in daily practices that in turn open up other opportunities for being empowered and empowering others.

Reflector

Think about your recent practice. In what ways have you helped other healthcare professionals to gain some sense of emancipation in their work? In what ways has anyone offered you the means to feel liberation of some sort in your work? If the outlook is bleak and few emancipatory events happen where you work, you may find that reflective practice heightens your awareness for liberating change for you and your colleagues.

In summary, critical knowledge is potentially liberating for individuals and groups of people, when they realize that they may be living under systematically entrenched misunderstandings about themselves and their social situations. As people and clinicians, healthcare professionals are subject to oppressive social structures, which can be transformed through critical reflection and action, the results of which constitute critical knowledge.

Knowledge and human interests

Jurgen Habermas, a prominent philosopher and sociologist, expounded a compelling critical theory of knowledge and human interests. These ideas are central to how I formulated the three kinds of reflection. My description of Habermas' ideas is derived from some of his work (Habermas 1972) and from other writers who have supported his work (Mezirow 1981; Fay 1987).

As a critical theorist, Habermas argued that human knowledge could be categorized as technical, practical and emancipatory, based on primary cognitive interests. He suggested that these areas are 'knowledge-constitutive interests', because they determine what humans count as important knowledge. He based this on his reasoning that humans have constructed experience socially, and that knowledge and social existence represent identifiable human interests. In other words, he claimed that knowledge and how we judge it to be 'truth' (epistemology) is constructed according to the sense we make of our existence and how we live socially (ontology). He argued that these interests in knowledge are based on aspects of social existence, such as work, human interactions and power relationships. He connected technical interests to work, practical interests to interaction and emancipatory interests to power. I have adopted the categorizations of these interests to name the types of reflection described in this book.

Technical interest and work

In Habermas' view, technical interest in work creates 'instrumental action' through which people control and manipulate their environments. This means that people act in accordance with technical rules to generate empirical knowledge, which can be proven to be correct or incorrect according to the rules of the scientific method. The empirical–analytical sciences have been developed to assist in understanding technical interests relating to work. These sciences are identified readily by their use of quantitative research methods, which allow them to generalize results and predict future tendencies for similar effects and outcomes to occur. For healthcare professionals, this means that technical interest is associated with task-related competence, such as clinical procedures. There is an increasing call in healthcare for evidence as a basis for better practice, and many of the work practices that need to be improved require technical interest using objective and systematic lines of inquiry, so this interest fits well with technical reflection, to be described later.

Practical interest and interaction

Practical interest involves human interaction, or 'communicative action', which involves reciprocal expectations about behaviour, which are defined and understood by the people concerned. Social norms, or sets of expectations for behaviour, are created over time by people who are in consensus as to what is expected in certain situations. The social norms are enforced through sanctions, which ensure that people recognize and honour their responsibilities in reciprocal behaviour. If this sounds complex, think of it in a healthcare context, where communicative action translates to something as familiar as the communication patterns that are set up by clinicians with other people. For example, the ways in which you communicate may differ between people – you may communicate in a certain way with relatives in a waiting room and in a different way with colleagues at the unit desk.

Practical interest in communicative action requires understanding it according to the people involved. Its main intentions are to describe and explain human interaction, so this kind of interest is mediated through language, which describes and explains the area of interest. Previously I referred to this kind of knowledge as interpretive knowledge, because it intends to understand human interaction through understanding the meaning of experience. Practical interests abound in healthcare and they can be reflected on systematically through practical reflection, described later in this chapter.

Emancipatory interest and power

Emancipatory interest is rooted in power and creates 'transformative action'. It involves the interpretive elements as described previously, because people interpret themselves in terms of their roles and social obligations. However, the main intentions of emancipatory interest are motivated by 'transformative action' which seeks to provide liberation from forces which limit people's rational control of their lives. These forces are so influential and taken for granted that they give people the strong impression that they are beyond their control.

The modes of inquiry for exploring and critiquing emancipatory interests associated with power are the critical social sciences, such as critical forms of sociology, politics and feminism. Critical theorists suggest that people must become conscious 'of how an ideology reflects and distorts moral, social and political reality and what material and psychological factors influence and sustain the false consciousness which it represents – especially reified powers of domination' (Mezirow 1981: 145). The kind of radical critique suggested by Mezirow is necessary for healthcare professionals as they examine the effects of power in their work settings and how situations become entrenched and taken for granted, and continue to constrain work relationships and practices.

Thus, I have adopted the label of 'emancipatory reflection' to uncover and potentiate emancipatory interests at work.

In summary, in this book I have chosen to refer to three types of reflection, which are derived from Habermas' technical, practical and emancipatory 'knowledge-constitutive interests'. This is not a novel decision, as similar approaches have been taken in education and research. Habermas connected technical interests to work, practical interests to human interaction and emancipatory interests to power. Technical interest in work creates 'instrumental action' through which people control and manipulate their environments. Practical interest creates human interaction or 'communicative action', which involves reciprocal expectations about behaviour, defined and understood by the people involved. Emancipatory interest is rooted in power and creates 'transformative action' through which people can free themselves from forces which limit their rational control of their lives. In the next section, I connect Habermas' 'knowledge-constitutive interests' to technical, practical and emancipatory reflection.

Table 3.1 may help you to distinguish the features of each paradigm according to the cognitive interests related to the kind of reflection, the aspects of social existence, and the action and learning involved.

Three types of reflection

Healthcare professionals engaged in daily practice have the advantage of living their practice, in that they have opportunities to look every day at their practice to learn from it. When healthcare professionals reflect on what they do, they can make sense of their practice, and imagine and/or bring about changes. The type of change they desire might direct the type of reflection they use.

Table 3.1 Three paradigms of knowledge with associated cognitive interests, aspects of social existence, action and learning involved

	Paradigm of knowledge		
	Empirical	Interpretive	Critical
Cognitive interests related to the kind of reflection	Technical	Practical	Emancipatory
Aspect of social existence	Work	Interaction	Power
Action involved	Instrumental	Communicative	Transformative
Learning involved	Task-related competence	Interpersonal	Transformative

In this section I highlight the advantages and limitations of technical, practical and emancipatory reflection. I also suggest that each type is as important as the others and that a type or combination of types may be used according to the requirements of a clinical situation. Because each of these ways of reflecting is important, I have devoted a chapter to each of them in this book. All I am intending to do in this section is to give you a brief introduction to the individual features of technical, practical and emancipatory reflection.

Technical reflection

The influence of the scientific model on empirical knowledge is apparent in daily practice. Many innovations and evidence-based adaptations in healthcare have been possible because of empirical knowledge, which is gained through empirical research and technical reflection.

The scientific method and rational, deductive thinking and reflection allow you to generate and validate empirical knowledge through rigorous means, so that you can be assured that work procedures are based on scientific reasoning. If clinical questions and issues are complex, as they tend to be when they are related to competency in practice, technical reflection may accompany empirical research projects, which are based on reliability, validity, and control and manipulation of variables. The technical reflection thus instigated will produce objective data that can be quantified to demonstrate the degree of statistical significance in cause and effect relationships. Technical reflection allows you to adapt and improve work procedures. You may also be able to predict likely outcomes for similar procedures. Technical reflection helps you to improve your instrumental action through technical control and manipulation in devising and improving procedural approaches to your work.

Although technical reflection offers a great deal of important knowledge in relation to providing evidence for the competency of work practices and procedures, by itself it will not be sufficient to interpret the meaning of what it is like to exist and work in settings that rely on making sense of interpersonal communication patterns and behaviours. Technical reflection by itself will not assist you in understanding the social interactions and consensual norms that govern the communication of the people undertaking and receiving the procedures, because it does not have an interest in human interaction and communicative action. Also, technical reflection by itself will not raise your awareness of power relationships between the givers and receivers of procedures and it will not provide a radical critique of the unexamined assumptions about social, economic, historical and cultural influences that underlie the instrumental action in procedural activities, because it does not have an interest in power and transformative action.

Technical reflection methods and processes are explained in detail in Chapter 4.

Practical reflection

Interpretation for description and explanation are the key outcomes of practical reflection, which focuses on human interaction in social existence. Communicative action in healthcare relates to shared communication of norms and expectations.

Practical reflection offers a means of making sense of human interaction. Through the medium of language, practical reflection helps you to understand the interpersonal basis of human experiences and offers you the potential for creating knowledge, which interprets the meaning of lived experience, context and subjectivity. It also offers you the potential for change, based on your raised awareness of the nature of a wide range of communicative matters pertaining to your healthcare profession.

However, practical reflection will not offer you the objective means to observe and analyse work procedures through a scientific method, because it does not have an interest in instrumental action. Also, practical reflection will not offer you a radical critique of the constraining forces and power influences within healthcare settings. The reason for this is that, although practical reflection can raise awareness through insights into communicative action, it does not have transformative action as its primary concern.

Practical reflection methods and processes are explained in detail in Chapter 5.

Emancipatory reflection

Emancipatory reflection involves human interaction, but its focus is on how people interpret themselves politically in terms of their roles and social obligations. Emancipatory reflection leads to 'transformative action', which seeks to free practitioners from assumptions and oppressive forces which limit them and their practice.

Emancipatory reflection provides you with a systematic means of critiquing the power relationships in your workplace and offers you raised awareness and a new sense of informed consciousness to bring about positive social and political change. Emancipatory reflection also offers you the potential to identify your own misguided and firmly held perceptions of yourself and your roles, to bring about positive change. The process of emancipatory reflection for change is praxis. Praxis in healthcare offers clinicians the means for change through collaborative processes that analyse and challenge existing forces and distortions brought about by dominating effects of power in human interaction.

Even though emancipatory reflection provides a critique of power in your work setting and relationships, it will not offer you a central focus on the technical interest of procedures at work, because it does not have an abiding and primary interest in instrumental action. Also, even though it begins with analyses of social interactions and consensual norms that govern human communication, emancipatory reflection is more concerned with examining the distortions that occur in communicative action than it is with generating a rich description of the meaning of human experience as it is lived by people involved in the practice of a healthcare profession.

Emancipatory reflection methods and processes are explained in detail in Chapter 6.

Choosing a type of reflection

No type of reflection is better than another; each has its own value for different purposes. This is the same as saying that no one form of knowledge is superior to another. For example, empirical knowledge was once valued over other types. For a long time, healthcare professionals thought they had to imitate the medical model and the scientific method in the way they thought about and researched their work. As a consequence of dominant scientific approaches, a culture developed which included specific traditions, such as the use of objective language in conversations and professional notes, and reductionist approaches to people requiring specific attention to affected body parts. Added to this was a strong belief that the only kind of research that was useful and valid was quantitative, because it involved prediction, control, numbers and statistics, which were seen to serve medical practice well. Some healthcare professionals have 'moved on' from the days of medical domination and scientific rationality, but many more may not be aware of the other choices they can make in making sense of their practice.

All kinds of knowledge can be generated through reflection, and healthcare professionals can benefit from a range of reflective processes. The first set of questions you should ask yourself in choosing a specific type or combination of types of reflection consist of: 'What do I want to know through reflection?' 'Why do I want to know it?' 'What questions will stimulate and guide my reflections and lead me to the answers I am seeking?' 'Is my primary focus on work procedures, human interaction or power relationships, or a combination of these interests?'

In this section, I described the features of technical, practical and emancipatory reflection. Finding a balance for using types of knowledge and reflection is important, because knowledge exists for all sorts of purposes and the reflective means healthcare professionals use will depend on what they need to achieve. The categories of reflection are artificial and contrived for convenience – they do not exist in isolation from one another and they are not mutually exclusive. Remember this as you read on through this book, so that your choices can be informed by broader considerations than choosing one type of reflection over another. If you can develop a reflective consciousness based on balance and context, it will serve you well in deciding how to reflect on any issue which presents itself in your practice.

Being human as a model of healthcare

In this section, I offer a model of caring which values the ordinariness of being human and of sharing those qualities in providing healthcare for other humans. Ordinariness as genuine, uncomplicated presencing and relating in human-to-human care can be used in daily combination with reflection to enhance knowledge, skills and humanity in your practice.

Author's reflection

I was working in my back garden moving uprooted plants from one part of the garden to a newly prepared patch, when I found myself thinking about this book. I am a 'rough and tumble' type of gardener – I absorb myself totally in the work, 'head down, bum up', like my granny and mother before me, making a lot of difference in a short time. I live in a subtropical area in northern New South Wales, Australia, where there is plenty of rain and sunshine, so my 'slap happy' gardening methods usually pay off splendidly despite minimum horticultural know-how.

I love metaphors for making sense of my life and the garden is a rich bed of reflection. For example, some people in my work life have been sweet-smelling violets, but their friendship has been short-lived and fragile, while others are roses with good looks, fragrance and hardiness, but their thorns have cut deeply. My favourite colleagues have been less showy flowers, always resilient and growing in impossible places in all kinds of conditions, with enough colour and cheer to make my heart glad. The metaphor goes on and on, but you get the idea.

So, I was working in my garden, thinking about my life in retirement and how I now have the time and space to relax and to just 'be' and reflect, and my thoughts turned to this book. I thought about the chapters and how the book would be different from the previous edition – for example, in broadening its focus to all healthcare professionals. Extra to that though, I realized as I bent over the garden patch transplanting a frangipani into a hastily dug hole, that this book needed to be more explicit in connecting the personal to the professional. I realized that my personal theory of practice is that self-work permeates professional work and that the more I understand and enhance myself, the more I can offer to others in my workplace. That is when I decided to insert these author's reflections into the text, so I can share with you something of my own evolution to date as a human being.

As soon as I thought of making more personal–professional connections in this book, my thoughts turned to Carmen. I remembered her walking into my office, requesting PhD supervision. A year previously, she had been gravely ill in a local hospital and had requested to go home into the care of her husband, to die. She did not die then, rather she underwent an incredible recovery, which she wanted to describe in a reflective topical autobiographical project (RTA). As an artist, Carmen depicted her experience of living with cancer in paint and crayon images and she reflected deeply on her experiences of the biomedical and complementary options open to her. Her PhD was awarded posthumously in May 2009. Carmen's complex and deeply personal experience of illness, recovery, illness and dying are intensely instructive for healthcare professionals (Zammit 2008).

Carmen came to my mind as I worked in the garden, because I was pondering her central dilemma – that she did not feel a deep connection with the biomedical and complementary healthcare professionals, who attended to her disease, but not to her personhood. That's when I decided to include a model of human care in this book, to honour Carmen's memory and to offer something to help other people like Carmen, who want to feel acknowledged as a human when they receive healthcare. My own PhD project explored the phenomenon of ordinariness as shared humanity, which is being human when caring for people. Even though the project was undertaken with nurses, it has a generic appeal as a middle range theory to enable any healthcare professional to be more humanly real and genuine in interactions with clients.

The idea of researching the phenomenon of ordinariness in nursing originated from discussions with my research supervisor, Professor Alan Pearson (1988), who made some clinical observations in his own nursing practice that when he joked and generally took time to interact on an ordinary human level with clients, the experience of nursing was enhanced for his clients and himself. At that time, Alan was the Dean of Faculty of Nursing at Deakin University, in Victoria, Australia, leading an enthusiastic academic and clinical team in nursing practice, education and research. I was happy to take on the project of ordinariness, because in my Master of Education research (Taylor 1988) I also found that when I asked women in a postnatal ward to describe the midwives who were most effective in caring for them, they described those midwives who were 'just themselves'. The mothers differentiated between those midwives who they perceived as 'professional' in a detached way, and the midwives who were 'ordinary' human beings, in addition to being clinically effective.

The full details of the project can be procured in the thesis document by contacting Deakin University (Taylor 1991), as the book on my PhD project is now out of print. Essentially, I explored nurse–patient relationships, using a phenomenological approach, to uncover the everyday human qualities and activities of ordinary humanness in nursing. The *Oxford Dictionary* defines 'ordinary' as 'the most commonly found or attested', and in relation to people, ordinary is 'typical of a particular group, average'. Therefore, the sense of ordinary, for both language and people, is that of shared qualities, not as mediocrity, as you might first think when you hear the word 'ordinariness'.

After observing nursing encounters, interviewing nurses and patients, and keeping my personal–professional journal, eight major aspects of being human emerged from the research approach: facilitation; fair play; familiarity; family; favouring; feelings; fun; and friendship. Each of the aspects has subsets, or qualities and activities, comprising its identity. The key to finding humanness within the aspects is in locating their inner nature, and through the phenomenological analysis of the practice stories, I saw that within facilitation there is allowingness; within fair play there is straightforwardness; within familiarity there is self-likeness; within family there is homeliness; within favouring there is favourableness; within feelings there is in-tuneness; within fun there is lightheartedness and within friendship there is connectedness.

As these eight aspects describe the nature and effects of being human in caring contexts, they can be applied to any healthcare situation where there is resonance with the ideas and attempts to honour humanness in genuine human-to-human care.

Facilitation and allowingness

Facilitation refers to enabling qualities and activities, whereby a person makes certain challenges being experienced by another person easier to face. Some qualities and activities of facilitation in healthcare include: appreciating skilful care; appreciating help; facilitating independence; facilitating learning; facilitating coping; facilitating comfort; facilitating acceptance of body image changes; facilitating changes; calming fears; building trust; giving confidence; and allowing the experience to unfold.

Healthcare professionals are registered to practise as competent practitioners, and their professional knowledge and skills are expected and generally appreciated daily by clients in caring contexts. Healthcare professionals are able to work skilfully, informed by the ever-growing knowledge base derived from their professional education and their clinical experiences. Therefore, clients place their trust in healthcare professionals to care for them skilfully.

Independence is claimed and assisted. To be independent assumes freedom from control of some sort. In healthcare, clients can claim their independence and professionals can help themselves towards it. Clients may be keen to develop their own level of independence and to express themselves as individuals. The need for independence varies according to the unique situation of each client. Healthcare professionals can work with clients to find a balance between helping and not helping, so that clients are able to resume some degree of autonomous action as soon as possible.

Learning is important for clients and healthcare professionals. Clients need to be invested in their learning, because it gives them the knowledge and skills they need to cope with the effects of illness. Healthcare professionals can give clients the tools of their freedom, by making learning easier. They can make learning easier by the ways in which they bring their knowledge, skills and humanity to the teaching context. Teaching is a process of person-to-person communication, through which important information and skills are shared with clients, to enable them to cope better with their changed life circumstances.

The stress of illness and disability, to varying degrees, can distort a client's ability to manage daily activities. For some clients, the road back to where they were originally, or to a renewed health status, represents a major journey. The path back to optimal well-being is made easier to traverse when clients learn how to cope with their changed life circumstances. Healthcare professionals can make coping easier for clients by the way they encourage them to become proactive in finding their own level of independence and in making reasoned choices amongst lifestyle and treatment alternatives.

For clients, a sense of comfort is integral to the everyday experience of being human. Being relatively free from various forms of psychological and physiological discomforts is a welcome relief from the changes to usual life patterns caused by illness. Healthcare professionals can make the attainment of comfort easier for clients by 'being there' authentically, assisting them with their daily activities and providing judicious emotional support, sensitive to the unique circumstances of each client. Attending carefully to physical comfort measures often has the effect of attending simultaneously to the client's emotional comfort.

Sometimes recovery from an illness means changes in a person's usual body structures and functions. Whereas some alterations in the body's physiological functions may be unapparent, visible anatomical alterations present unique challenges to clients. For example, waking from surgery and getting accustomed to living without a body part is managed by each person in his or her own way. Healthcare professionals can be present authentically for clients, to make the acceptance of an altered body image easier. There is no prescriptive approach to facilitating acceptance of clients' body image changes; rather, it is something which unfolds with patience and sensitivity, according to the unique circumstances of the people involved.

As part of their treatment, clients are often confronted with the necessity of making considerable changes in their lifestyles. Making changes in life patterns is difficult, especially when patterns have been developed over long periods of time. Healthcare professionals can make changes easier for clients by encouraging them to understand the need for treatment and to choose to persist with it, in order to find ways of incorporating new regimes into their daily life. Changes begin with clients, because their cooperation is integral to making changes successfully.

Illness and hospitalization may create many fears for clients, who cope in various ways. Fears may be real or imagined, relatively small or overwhelming, but they are experienced and they persist until they can be alleviated in some way. Healthcare professionals can alleviate fears through careful, age-appropriate explanations, general talk and company, in whatever amounts and combinations that suit a particular client's needs.

Clients submit themselves to hospitalization and the uncertainty that it often entails and their new experiences present challenges, especially that of putting their trust in healthcare professionals who are relative strangers. Part of a client's recovery may be a reaffirmation of trust in themselves and other people. Healthcare professionals can help to build trust by 'being there' authentically with clients daily, assisting them through the stages of their illness experiences, and sharing with them as people. Healthcare professionals and clients can build trust through mutual self-disclosure, so that by showing each other something of themselves as humans, they begin to acknowledge their shared humanness and to trust each other.

Healthcare professionals can give clients confidence to resume their usual lives. There is no singular approach that functions routinely to give confidence, rather giving confidence is something that is orchestrated spontaneously in the daily round of activities, whenever healthcare professionals and clients interact with one another.

Experiences of life unfold daily for healthcare professionals and clients. Each day is faced for what it brings forth, and people react to things and interpret them in various ways. Being relatively free from preconceptions of what might happen and how clients might need to be treated does not apply to standard technical procedures, which are a part of the care of each client. Each client requires a certain standard of care in relation to his or her total management and that must be attended to, as necessary. However, when it comes to personal preferences and subjective experiences, as reflected in spontaneous communication and lifestyle choices, minimal prejudgement is needed of how clients 'should' feel and behave.

Allowingness is the essential human nature embodied in facilitation. Allowingness creates the potential for clients and healthcare professionals to help themselves, by providing some guidance and support until such a time, if at all, that clients feel able to take over their own daily life business. Allowingness is being considerate of the other person's needs to be independent and dignified; it helps quietly and carefully, always attentive to the cues within the other person, that suggest a preparedness to resume increasingly autonomous thoughts and actions. Allowingness is an essence of being human, by relating to another human through sensitive helping.

Fair play and straightforwardness

Fair play refers to the sense of reasonableness we possess as humans, through which we are forthright in saying what we feel we have to say, knowing that the least we can do, even partially, is to tolerate frustrating elements in others that we recognize in ourselves. Some qualities and activities of fair play include straight talking and tolerating one another's humanness respectfully.

Speaking messages frankly and clearly occurs between healthcare professionals and clients, in situations in which one person has something to say for the benefit of the other, even though the listener may have some difficulty in hearing it. Straight talking is returned in kind to the speaker, because the controversial nature of the talk creates a reaction, which also needs to be expressed. Healthcare professionals and clients expect to 'take turns' at being both speaker of and listener to straight talk. Although it risks hurt feelings, it can 'clear the air' between people and allows frank and honest dialogue when matters are contentious.

The more time healthcare professionals and clients take to get to know one another in the course of day-to-day events, the more they begin to recognize and tolerate respectfully human features in each other. They realize that the so-called 'roles' of client and healthcare professional are not scripted strictly and that each person can take the opportunity to 'ad lib' should the mood and the moment dictate. For instance, clients are not always long-suffering, and healthcare professionals are not always cheerful. Regardless of their roles in healthcare settings clients and healthcare professionals are 'only human'.

Straightforwardness is the essential human nature of fair play. It creates the potential for clients and healthcare professionals to speak to each other as frankly as possible, saying whatever it is that is in need of being said, at the same time tolerating each other's humanness respectfully. Straightforwardness is clear and concise in its delivery and generous in its intent; it speaks to the other to unblock impasses and puts the perceived focus of contention plainly on view, to trigger discussion. Straightforwardness is an essence of being human, by relating to another person through sensitive straight talking.

Familiarity and self-likeness

Familiarity refers to that sense we have of someone else, through the sense we have of ourselves, as individuals with a lifetime of experiences. Some qualities and activities of familiarity include: relating to one another's humanness; relating to the other's situation; acknowledging specialness in everyday situations; tolerating noisiness; relating to the client as a person; relating to the healthcare professional as person; relating to each other as people; relating to genuineness in people; equating with a sense of 'that's all;' recognizing the days on which everything seems to go wrong and being part of everyday life.

Healthcare professionals and clients can share a sense of what it is for them to be human themselves and how humanness might seem for someone else. Relating to one another's humanness creates a strong bond between healthcare professionals and clients, who reveal something of themselves to one another and sense an affinity as people living out their day-to-day lives in healthcare contexts.

Healthcare professionals and clients can begin to understand each other in relation to the unique circumstances in which they find themselves. When there is mutual respect, not only do healthcare professionals relate to clients' circumstances, but also clients can become aware of, and sensitive to, the healthcare professionals' circumstances as human beings in healthcare roles.

Both parties may begin to realize that there is specialness in the everyday activities in which they are engaged routinely together. Healthcare professionals can acknowledge the value of time spent with clients, while undertaking professional tasks and activities. Accomplishing daily tasks provides space and time for continuing dialogue and increased familiarity with clients.

On occasions, healthcare settings can be noisy with the traffic and clatter of everyday life, however, clients and healthcare professionals may seem to be oblivious to the noise, when they are intent on what they are doing, or when the noise is actually comfortable in a friendly, familiar sort of way.

Healthcare professionals can learn to relate to their clients as people, who are living their own particular lives and present circumstances within the context of a healthcare setting. Healthcare professionals can learn to value clients as people with a past, present and future as unique individuals, through relating to them respectfully as human beings.

Clients form opinions about and are able to relate to healthcare professionals as people. Some clients feel free and able to express how they feel about a particular healthcare professional as a person, whereas others simply acknowledge 'liking' or 'disliking' a professional with whom they have interacted.

Clients are able to recognize genuineness in healthcare professionals by differentiating professionals who are being 'real', honest and caring, from those professionals who are simply 'going through the motions' of enacting a detached professional role. A client may recognize that genuineness in a professional shows that this person 'gives a damn' and relates to their clients with genuine concern.

Healthcare professionals and clients coexist in healthcare settings and some of them appear to cease to notice the relative strangeness of what happens in the context, compared with their usual home surroundings and lifestyles. For example, taken for granted acceptance may show itself when clients adapt easily to having a healthcare professional perform an intimate procedure, by equating it with a sense of 'that's all'; or 'they are just doing their job.' The taken for granted acceptance is also exemplified by some healthcare professionals, whose relatively sophisticated technical and communicative skills are combined into sheer artistry, yet these professionals appear to be unselfconscious of themselves and their expertise. They express a sense of 'that's all' as 'its just part of my job!'

On some days, nothing seems to go well in life, and these days can happen in healthcare settings. Healthcare professionals need to be aware that on some days, even with high standards and continued attention to detail, things seem to go wrong. Professionals and clients are immersed in the daily context of healthcare settings, which are busy places in which people move to and fro, continuing their interpersonal communications and enacting their own agendas within the healthcare culture. Even on days when things seem to go wrong, regardless of their personal plights and emotions, healthcare professionals need to realize that they can make their way authentically through the temporary chaos by 'in the moment' human communication.

Self-likeness is the essential human nature of familiarity. People see themselves mirrored, to some degree, in other people. Self-likeness creates the potential for clients and healthcare professionals to understand the humanness of themselves in others, sharing an affinity as humans together, bonded by the commonality of their ordinary human existence. Self-likeness is the glue of oneness, wherein people share a sense of togetherness, regardless of a vicissitude of differences; it is a source of recognition of being human, as a sense of the ultimate sameness of all people and things. Self-likeness is an essence of being human, through recognition of another human and sensitive relating.

Family and homeliness

Family refers to the sense of home we have within ourselves, which binds us to people with whom we have blood ties or special affinities. Some qualities and activities of family include: acknowledging the relevance of family affiliations to the person; expressing 'family-like' ties; appreciating a 'home-like' atmosphere and preparing to go home.

A healthcare setting is a separate world from the time and space of home realities, however family affiliations can be recognized and valued within everyday dialogue between healthcare professionals and clients. In keeping family affiliations paramount, professionals and clients can remind each other of their identities as people and 'meet each other in the middle', to bridge the gap between the 'artificiality' of the healthcare environment and the 'naturalness' of home. Acknowledging the relevance of family and home varies for different people and their respective affiliations.

Home is ever present in the day-to-day dialogue between healthcare professionals and clients. Professionals encourage clients to align themselves with home, and together they negotiate usual home routines associated with activities of daily living into the healthcare setting as often as possible.

Sometimes the sense of family is reflected in special affinities between healthcare professionals and clients, who become so close to one another that the relationship is best expressed as a 'family-like' tie. For example, a client may say of a professional, 'He was like a brother to me.'

Healthcare settings are structured and professional, however they can allow for relaxed interactions, creating a 'home-like' context into which other health professionals and non-family members come as guests and 'visitors'.

Even though healthcare settings may attempt to be 'home-like', given the circumstances of people being uprooted from their usual life contexts by illness or other misfortune, they cannot and do not attempt to replace home as the most treasured place for people to be. Healthcare is geared towards helping people to return to their homes, if it is humanly possible. Clients prepare to go home with varying states of anticipation, depending on how they feel they will cope with their particular circumstances. Some clients realize that they will never go home again – for example, an elderly care unit may need to become the less favoured but necessary option.

Homeliness creates the potential for clients and healthcare professionals to develop close interpersonal relationships that encompass the perspectives of people as family. Homeliness is sharing common understandings with people, and in so doing accepting a share of their joys and pains, which are integral to closer human relationships. Homeliness is an essence of being human, by relating to that person through sensitive family-like bonding.

Favouring and favourableness

Favouring refers to the approval we give to other people and ourselves for commendable qualities, which remind us of our essential nature as human beings. Some qualities and activities of favouring include approving commendable human qualities and enjoying statements of appreciation.

Clients and healthcare professionals recognize and approve commendable human qualities in each other, such as goodness, niceness, loveliness, friendliness, helpfulness, kindness, caring and gentleness. These qualities are often expressed without further elaboration, as though extra words will not say more. The expressions of approval belie an affinity of liking and appreciation between clients and healthcare professionals, and in affirming these qualities within others, each reaffirms the same qualities within themselves. In other words, I can recognize and respect goodness and niceness in another person when I know I am basically a good and nice person.

Healthcare professionals work daily with people, doing their jobs to the best of their abilities and not expecting to receive statements of appreciation in return. When they do receive a compliment, however, professionals accept it, possibly shyly, but always with some degree of appreciation.

Favourableness reminds us of our own commendable qualities by seeing them in other people, as a mirror of our essential nature as human beings. Favourableness creates the potential for clients and healthcare professionals to give approval to other people and themselves, and in so doing to magnify the attractive aspects of themselves. Favourableness is seeing beauty in people at the inside level; it recognizes everyday human qualities that defy adequate description, because we know these qualities exist and how they manifest themselves. Favourableness is an essence of being human, by relating to another human through sensitive favouring.

Feelings and in-tuneness

Feelings refer to the way we sense ourselves in relation to people and things: sometimes as feeling high, sometimes as feeling low, sometimes as feeling somewhere in between. Some qualities and activities of feelings include acknowledging the polarity of human feelings and expressing those feelings.

In their daily lives in healthcare settings, healthcare professionals and clients can learn to acknowledge the polarity of their human feelings. Depending on what is happening for each individual, professionals and clients can acknowledge and respect the presence, in themselves and others, of the full range of human feelings, including being happy or sad, being in comfort or pain, being relaxed or agitated, being calm or in fear and being angry or content.

Having feelings, and actually expressing them, can be two different things. Healthcare professionals and clients can learn to give voice to their feelings in relation to all sorts of things, about whatever is of interest to them, according to the particular situations in which they find themselves. When there is mutual respect and acceptance as human beings, professionals and clients can come to understand that there is full licence to express the polarity of their feelings and avail themselves of these opportunities.

In-tuneness is clearing away the debris of rationality, to face up to, and embrace, the rawness of emotions, which when expressed unblock the streams of human reactivity and cause our life energies to flow a little easier. In-tuneness is an essence of being human, by relating to another human through sensitive expressions of feeling.

Fun and lightheartedness

Fun refers to a sense of merriment which lightens our daily lives and reacquaints us with the child within us. Fun includes enjoying a sense of humour.

Healthcare professionals and clients can exhibit their enjoyment of a sense of humour by laughing, joking, cheekiness and general happiness. A sense of humour can permeate a healthcare setting to the extent that even people in pain and distress appreciate a well-placed light word or joke. It is as though humour softens the hard realities of people's circumstances and provides a means of levity, albeit temporarily, above the inevitability of certain ultimate tragedies. Humour is always shared, never imposed. Humour is always sensitive to the other's situation and reaches across the gap of the singular existence of healthcare professionals and clients, to seal their common humanity with a shared sense of merriment.

Lightheartedness is sharing our sense of fun. It creates the potential for clients and healthcare professionals to express themselves through humour. Lightheartedness seeks to aerate the lead ball of life and turn it into a bright balloon. It is an essence of being human, by relating to another human through sensitive humouring.

Friendship and connectedness

Friendship refers to knowing people well enough to regard them with affection. Some qualities and activities of friendship include acknowledging the importance of company and talking, expressing affection and liking and taking time to know one another.

Healthcare professionals and clients spend time together in healthcare settings, and they can acknowledge the value of 'being there' for one another for companionship and support. Clients value the non-instrumental time healthcare professionals spend with them. Healthcare professionals can learn to understand that sometimes company and talking are the most they can provide, when nothing else can be done.

Some healthcare professionals and clients know each other so well that they feel and express affection and liking for each other. Affection comes from catching glimpses of each other as people, whose many human similarities far outweigh their differences in terms of professional knowledge and skills. Affection and liking towards one another can extend past the world of healthcare to connections with each other after the period of care. Close ties with clients creates some personal emotional risks and vulnerabilities associated with closeness, especially as some clients will continue to be readmitted to the healthcare setting until they eventually succumb to their disease in death.

Some healthcare settings are conducive for people coming to know one another well. Depending on the time span and frequency of interactions, clients and healthcare professionals can get to know one another to varying degrees. The time clients and professionals spend together is interrupted, over the course of a day's treatments and care. As paid workers, healthcare professionals come to the healthcare setting and go home daily, take days off and go on holidays, and clients recover and go home, are transferred elsewhere, or die. Even so, in some healthcare settings, it is possible for healthcare professionals and clients to get to know one another well as human beings.

Time and opportunity create differences in the ways healthcare professionals and clients are able to get to know one another, however, intensive efforts can be made to shorten the introductory periods of relationships, so that people get to know one another as well as possible, in whatever time is available. For healthcare professionals there is much to know about clients, not only about their experiences of their illnesses, but also about who and how they are as people with social networks and individual hopes and fears.

Connectedness is sensing ourselves as friends. It creates the potential for clients and healthcare professionals to know one another well enough to regard each other with affection. Connectedness is recognizing friendly aspects in other people and coming in closer to get to know them. It takes time to get to know the other person, through keeping company and talking. Connectedness is an essence of being human, by relating to another human through sensitive liking.

Summary

In this section, I described a model of humanness in healthcare, by outlining some key ideas in my PhD research, made generic to any healthcare professional. Ordinariness is the shared affinity we have as humans, which can permeate healthcare and give essential humanness to our existing knowledge and skills. The key to finding humanness and being human in healthcare is in locating and embodying its inner nature, that is, within facilitation there is allowingness; within fair play there is straightforwardness; within familiarity there is self-likeness; within family there is homeliness; within favouring there is favourableness; within feelings there is in-tuneness; within fun there is lightheartedness and within friendship there is connectedness.

Like all other humans, healthcare professionals are actually quite extraordinary in their ordinary humanness. This humanness is not, as might be first thought, a small and inconsequential thing. The potentiality of human nature is an empowering force for healthcare professionals and clients, and for people generally.

Healthcare professionals and clients are special in their human uniqueness, a phenomenon often forgotten, or taken for granted, in the familiarity of everyday embodied existence in healthcare settings. Healthcare professionals and clients are the same in their humanity and it is this sameness that transcends any apparent differences they might have as individuals. The generative force of humanness can be reclaimed, simply by the awareness, valuing and exercising of it.

Aspects of ordinariness such as facilitation, fair play, familiarity, family, favouring, feelings, fun and friendship can have advantageous effects. Healthcare professionals and clients can sense an affinity as humans and they negotiate the illness experience together through their human qualities of allowingness, straightforwardness, self-likeness, homeliness, favourableness, in-tuneness, lightheartedness and connectedness. The ordinariness of being human is sophisticated in its simplicity. The shared human qualities of healthcare professionals and clients have within them the generative source of humanness, which is the ability to care for, and about, one another.

Summary

In this chapter I began by describing the types of reflection which can be used in any combination to help you identify and work through your practice issues. Healthcare practice involves knowledge, skills and humanity and all three components need to be present before you can claim to be a safe, effective and empathic practitioner. Being a 'well-rounded' person and practitioner takes a lifetime of reflection, insights and adaptations, and even then there is still more to learn.

Technical, practical and emancipatory reflection will help you identify issues and constraints to improve your procedural work and interpersonal communications and will also help you to understand and be freed from power issues in your workplace. However, unless you make it a particular focus of your continued attention, you may not consider a relationship basic to your work – that of your therapeutic relationship with the clients in your care. Human interactions are fundamental to healthcare. Being human as a healthcare professional accentuates the opportunities for creating genuine person-to-person interactions in which the shared qualities of humanity are enhanced, such as in facilitation, fair play, familiarity, family, favouring, feelings, fun and friendship.

Key points

- When potentially complex phenomena are in focus, structures for thinking, such as theories, models and categories can be used gainfully.
- Empirical knowledge comes from technical reflection, interpretive knowledge comes from practical reflection and critical knowledge comes from emancipatory reflection.
- Empirical knowledge is generated and tested through 'the scientific method' and outcomes are achieved mainly through rational deductive thinking processes, which move systematically from broad to focused inferences.
- People are the focus of interpretive knowledge, because this form of knowledge features people's perceptions of their life experiences and their ability to communicate them, based on their interpersonal

understanding through attention to lived experience, context and subjectivity.

- Critical knowledge is derived from some key ideas in critical social science, such as false consciousness, hegemony, reification, emancipation and empowerment.
- Habermas connected technical interests to work, practical interests to interaction and emancipatory interests to power, and these categorizations are adopted in this book to name technical, practical and emancipatory reflection.
- Work practices that need to be improved require technical interest using objective and systematic lines of inquiry, so this interest fits well with technical reflection.
- Practical interest involves human interaction, or 'communicative action', involving reciprocal expectations about behaviour, defined and understood by the people involved, so practical interests in healthcare can be reflected on systematically through practical reflection.
- Emancipatory interest is rooted in power and creates 'transformative action', so emancipatory reflection can uncover and potentiate emancipatory interests at work.
- Technical reflection helps you to improve your instrumental action through technical control and manipulation in devising and improving procedural approaches to your work.
- Practical reflection helps you to understand the interpersonal basis of human experiences and offers you the potential for creating knowledge by interpreting the meaning of lived experience, context and subjectivity, and the potential for change, based on raised awareness of the nature of a wide range of communicative matters pertaining to healthcare.
- Emancipatory reflection leads to 'transformative action', which seeks to free you from taken-for-granted assumptions and oppressive forces, which limit you and your practice, by critiquing the power relationships in your workplace and offering you raised awareness and a new sense of informed consciousness to bring about positive social and political change.
- No type of reflection is better than another; each has its own value for different purposes.
- Ordinariness is the shared affinity we have as humans, which can permeate healthcare and give essential humanness to our existing knowledge and skills.
- Being human as a healthcare professional accentuates the opportunities for creating genuine person-to-person interactions in which the shared qualities of humanity are enhanced.

4 Technical reflection

Introduction

This chapter reviews information connected directly to technical reflection, including the reasons why this process is used for specific purposes and why it creates different outcomes in terms of knowledge of, and practical answers to, clinical problems. The relationships are explained between empirical knowledge and the scientific method, and how technical reflection fits with these ideas. The connections between technical reflection and evidence-based practice are described and you will find that the two processes are highly complementary. The chapter also describes the technical reflection process and examples of how technical reflection can be used by reflective healthcare professionals.

Technical reflection is important because it admits into the realms of reflection systematic thinking processes that are capable of bringing about sophisticated levels of argumentation, much needed to secure improvements in clinical policies and procedures. Therefore, this chapter justifies the value of technical reflection, based on its validity as a form of knowledge and its usefulness for clinical practice. I developed the process of technical reflection through an eclectic approach, borrowing ideas from Bandman and Bandman's (1995) view of scientific reasoning and the functions of critical thinkers, the features of critical thinking and thinkers described by van Hooft *et al.* (1995) and the problem-solving steps of the nursing process (Wilkinson 1996).

There are some important points to note before continuing. Although scientific reasoning and critical thinking have clear and distinctive purposes in generating and validating empirical knowledge, critical thinking also has wide applications and it may be helpful in any of the forms of reflection described in this book. However, critical thinking is most likely to be useful when you are raising questions in your practice about technicalities related to the form and usefulness of your work procedures and policies.

Also, remember that technical reflection may be used as a process in itself when you are working alone or with colleagues through observation and critical thinking, or it may be used in conjunction with research projects based on scientific reasoning that demand reliability, validity, and control and manipulation of variables. Alternatively, if a question posed as a reflective task is less complex and does not require a research project per se, technical reflection alone can lead to answers based on observation and sound arguments that incorporate rational aspects of critical thinking. It is also possible that technical reflection could become part of mixed methodology research, such as an action research project, using empirical methods to examine procedure 'X' as part of a larger collaborative group process. You need to exercise caution in determining whether a clinical problem is focused, and whether it can be resolved sufficiently by technical reflection alone. If there is any doubt as to whether the information generated is sufficient and effective, you may need to consider extending your reflections into a formal research project.

Review of previous ideas

Understanding the basis of technical reflection relies on information given earlier in this book, so you may choose to revisit Chapter 3. However, as background to this chapter, here are some essential points to tie the ideas firmly together.

Before you practise technical reflection it may help you to understand why this process is useful for specific purposes and why it creates specific outcomes in terms of knowledge of, and practical answers to, clinical problems. Integral to this understanding is the relationship between empirical knowledge and the scientific method, and how the process for technical reflection fits with these ideas. This section provides an epistemological explanation, which means that it describes how empirical knowledge is generated and validated.

Empirical knowledge rests on evidence from direct observation and is generated and tested through the 'scientific method'. Some scientists claim the scientific method is the only worthwhile method of knowledge generation and validation, because it has enjoyed long-lasting success in relation to technological innovations in areas such as medicine, psychology, physics, chemistry, biology, genetics, environmental sciences, engineering, architecture and so on. In fact, the proponents of the scientific method have such confidence in it that they claim empirical knowledge is the yardstick against which all other epistemological methods should be measured. The scientific method has been and continues to be very successful, because it uses strict criteria for setting up its inquiry and judging its truthfulness through rigorous and systematic measures including reliability, validity, and control and manipulation of variables.

Through the scientific method, data are quantified to demonstrate the degree of statistical significance in cause and effect relationships. In other words, information is converted into a numerical form, which can be measured and counted, so that it is possible to predict mathematically that the occurrence of a behaviour or experimental response is significant, and not just happening by chance. To achieve this kind of predictive ability, scientific knowledge is rendered as free as possible from the distorting influences of people, who may skew the results with their prejudices, intentions and emotions. To avoid subjectivity of this kind, empirical researchers demand objectivity, meaning they strive to ensure that there is no involvement of prejudices, intentions and emotions in the conduct of the project. In summary, the scientific method creates empirical knowledge, which can claim to be predictive and generalizable with some confidence that the conclusions are truthful, real, trustworthy and not just happening by chance.

The new or amended knowledge outcomes achieved by using the scientific method are mainly through rational deductive thinking processes, which move systematically from broad to focused inferences. Scientific reasoning refers to a certain kind of rational argument which underlies the scientific method. The scientific approach to reasoning is to state a problem, give a preliminary hypothesis setting out the expected relationships between variables, collect more facts in order to formulate a hypothesis, deduce further consequences, test those consequences, and finally apply the findings to confirm or disconfirm the hypothesis (Bandman and Bandman 1995). Scientific reasoning provides a systematic approach to working through complex problems in an objective manner designed to keep the inquirer on track and provide a means whereby other people can use a similar process to test whether the results can be repeated with the same results (replicated).

Reflector

Think of situations in which scientific reasoning is essential in your work. Why is it the best approach to problem-solving in these situations?

Critical thinking is the ability to think in a systematic and rational way. Scientific reasoning is aligned closely with critical thinking, in that the two processes share many characteristics and often lead to similar outcomes. Critical thinking is essential for safe clinical practice and, according to many authors, rationality is its first requirement (Bandman and Bandman 1995; van Hooft *et al*. 1995; Wilkinson 1996). However, some authors stress that critical thinking is not just about rationality and emotional detachment for intellectual 'purity'. Even though van Hooft *et al*. (1995: 6–7) are keen to define the first important element of critical thinking as rational thinking, they emphasize that it is practical as well as theoretical – that it is conducive to dialogue and that it includes empathy and sensitive perception. They also describe critical thinkers as committed, self-aware and sympathetic to the commitments of others. The addition of practicality, dialogue, empathy and sensitivity in critical thinking, and self-aware and altruistic features in critical thinkers, gives critical thinking a 'human touch' that elevates it above a pure exercise of scientific rationality as described previously. Even so, critical thinking borders on scientific reasoning, because of its emphasis on rationality and scientific reasoning.

Chapter 3 introduced the philosophy of Jurgen Habermas, whose ideas have been applied to practical areas such as curriculum (Mezirow 1981). Habermas is of interest to healthcare professionals because he had important things to say about the interests people have in their work, communication and power relations. When we consider technical reflection, we are focusing on what he had to say about work and procedures. In Habermas' view (1972), technical interest in work creates 'instrumental action' through which people control and manipulate their environments. This means that people work with intention, so that by keeping a 'hold' on situations they can achieve what they want. Therefore, people act in accordance with technical rules to generate empirical knowledge. In other words, they figure out the best ways of creating and following procedural steps in technical situations and claim that their results have been achieved through systematic and direct observation.

In healthcare professions, technical interest is associated with task-related competence, such as clinical procedures and policies. As you can see, this is another way of talking about empirical knowledge, rationality, the scientific method, critical thinking and problem-solving. The scientific method's influence on empirical knowledge is apparent in daily practice, because healthcare professionals have technical interest in their work. Many innovations and evidence-based adaptations in healthcare professions have been possible because of empirical knowledge, gained through empirical research, using processes described previously. Technical reflection fits into this discussion because it is a way for you to integrate ways of thinking, to allow you to adapt and improve procedures and policies. You may also be able to predict likely outcomes for similar procedures and improve many work practices through objective and systematic lines of inquiry.

Technical reflection fits well with evidence-based healthcare (Pearson *et al.* 1997; Shorten and Wallace 1997), which claims that practice needs to be based on research findings, rather than on rituals, traditions, whims and unfounded beliefs about what should or could be done in certain clinical situations. If you have been practising for some time now, you can probably remember how your profession's procedures have changed over time. At times, you may have wondered whether what you were doing was working at all and whether you had any technical justification for doing it. The evidence-based movement in healthcare professions is testing the validity of long-standing procedures and is replacing old untested and unproven approaches with newer research-based alternatives. Technical reflection is a systematic process for raising questions relating to procedures and policies providing strong argumentation based on scientific reasoning; therefore, it is highly complementary to evidence-based practice.

Practice story

Aliyah, a registered nurse with three years' experience post-graduation, began work in a rural hospital and noticed the tendency of the nurses working there to attend to all of the patients' hygiene needs by 10 a.m. After working in the hospital for two weeks, Aliyah prepared a presentation for the nurses' clinical meeting using the technical reflection process to question the soundness of, and necessity for, the procedure of nurses wanting to attend to patients' hygiene needs by this set time.

In the assessing and planning phase, Aliyah described the questionable procedure as 'attending to patients' hygiene needs by 10 a.m.'. She noticed that nurses showered, washed in bed or bathed patients, depending on their condition and willingness, between 7 a.m. and 10 a.m. The patients were clean and tidy by 10 a.m., ready for doctors' rounds, visitors and other procedures and appointments. Aliyah argued that the procedure was of questionable value because it served the purposes of the nurses and the ward routines, rather than the expressed wishes of individual patients. Her proposed amendment was that nurses undertake hygiene care at any time of the day according to patient preference, and cease the procedure of having all the hygiene needs completed by 10 a.m. Her preliminary hypothesis about the issue was: 'The problem of nurses needing to attend to patients hygiene needs by 10 a.m. is counterproductive and needs to be ceased, because hygiene needs will be better met if patients indicate their preferred method of hygiene at any time of the day that suits them'.

Aliyah explained that the procedure of meeting hygiene needs by 10 a.m. was associated with nurses' statements such as: 'We need to have everyone done by morning tea', 'There are five washes and two showers this morning', 'How many sponges have we got?' The words and language associated with meeting patients' hygiene needs by 10 a.m. related directly to getting the work done, on time. The 'misuse' of words and language was in the tendency to reduce patients to 'tasks to be done' and to approach hygiene needs as being specific to the needs of the ward, not the person: the patient. Aliyah argued that if the statements used commonly were looked at carefully, then nurses might identify their tendency to speak of patients' hygiene needs in terms of work to be done, on time. For example, differently stated the sentences could be: 'We need to attend to patients' hygiene needs, how and when they prefer', 'Five patients have indicated they want to have a wash and two patients have indicated they would like a shower, sometime today', 'How many people have indicated they would like a wash in bed?'

Critical friend response

Acting as a critical friend, I helped Aliyah to develop an argument by analysing the issues and assumptions operating in the situation, so she could present it to the nurses' clinical meeting.

Critical friend: *What arguments are made to support the continuation of meeting patients' hygiene needs by 10 a.m.?*

Aliyah: *Nurses who support the continuation of meeting all of the patients' hygiene needs by 10 a.m. argue that it helps patients to feel clean and comfortable and if patients are clean and comfortable then it will assist them in all aspects of their healing process.*

Critical friend: *What healthcare assumptions are these nurses making?*

Aliyah: *That all patients will be willing, cooperative and pleased to comply. However, the nurses may also want to continue the procedure, as it suits their purposes to have the bulk of the work done early in the day, and it also fits with the estab-lished ward routines of meal times, doctors' rounds, visitors and so on. Their premises are sound, that patients will feel clean and comfortable, and that will assist them in all aspects of their healing process.*

Critical friend: *Do these premises follow logically to provide sound conclusions?*

Aliyah: *No, not really, because the nurses' assumptions have not been made explicit. In addition, patients' healing processes can be facilitated by various means, and given that hygiene is only one of those important aspects, then it follows that it does not matter if the wash, shower or bath is taken after 10 a.m., indeed, it may be what the patient prefers. So, their inference is plausible in the sense that patients require hygiene care, but it is not plausible in specifying the time of day, as it does not necessarily follow that hygiene needs must be met by that time for the patients' benefit.*

Critical friend: *So, what are you arguing as an alternative procedure?*

Aliyah: *That although patients require hygiene care, this does not have to be attended to before 10 a.m., or at any particular*

> *time, because patients are usually in the best position to decide when they would prefer to have a wash, shower or bath. My assumptions for opposing the present procedure are that patients have a right to choose and nurses will be willing to comply with their wishes in relation to hygiene needs. I also challenge the previously unexpressed assumptions that nurses who continue the procedure are actually using it to serve their own purposes and to maintain the routines that meet the needs of a busy ward on a morning shift. Patients require hygiene care, but the time is unimportant, and patients who are able to do so are in the best position to decide when they would prefer to have a wash, shower or bath. One inference I am making is that if patients who are able are encouraged to decide when they want to have their hygiene needs met, then the nurses' work is in response to patients' needs, rather than the reverse. Another series of connected inferences I am making is that if the procedure is changed, then the ward work will not be compressed into three very busy hours in the morning, and if that is so, then nurses may find that the ward is less chaotic and that there is more time to spend with patients. If there is more time to spend with patients, then nurses and patients have the potential to create therapeutic relationships in which healing and well-being are promoted.*

Reflector

Think of a clinical procedure you have undertaken for some time now that you suspect is outmoded in some way. Why do you continue to perform that procedure in the same way, even though you suspect it is outmoded? Who needs to be convinced to change the procedure in your workplace?

The process of technical reflection

This section presents a process to assist you in using technical reflection in thinking about issues relating to a clinical procedure. There are many different methods for reflecting, and I understand that these methods may be used alone or in combination to assist you in letting your thoughts flow during reflective processes. Reflection does not have to be a solo effort. If you work better in groups, you can enlist a team or committee and go through reflective processes collaboratively. Technical reflection works well in groups and committees, when the process is used systematically and carefully. You may find that one 'run through' by yourself is a good idea, even if it just helps you get your thoughts together before a clinical meeting. Also, once you know how the process works, you can guide your colleagues through it, using this book as a reference.

The technical reflection process presented in this section encourages you to reflect on issues which require rational thinking for specific, manageable problems. As mentioned previously, if your clinical issues are especially complex and require protracted work to solve them, you may need to use technical reflection in conjunction with an empirical research design.

The outcomes of technical reflection can be immediate, if the process has been shared with, and the findings endorsed by, the key people who are in a position to influence and ratify healthcare practice. You may find that this process has many applications. For example, you could use technical reflection to think critically through your own practice issues, or it could be used in groups as a guide for a clinical policy and practice meeting agenda, as an outline for analysing technical issues in ward/unit clinical discussions, and/or as part of the methods of formal research. In whatever situations you use it, technical reflection has the potential for allowing you to think critically and reason scientifically, so that you can critique, adapt and improve procedures and policies. You may also be able to predict likely outcomes for similar procedures and improve many work practices through objective and systematic lines of inquiry.

I now present a process to assist you in using technical reflection in thinking about issues relating to a clinical procedure or policy. There are many different methods for reflecting, including writing, audiotaping, creative music, dancing and so on. These methods may be used alone or in combination to assist you in letting your thoughts flow during reflective processes.

Using the method(s) of your choice, consider the following questions. Respond as carefully as you can, making sure that you attend to every step along the way. Use as many words as necessary to explain your position thoroughly, but keep to the point, so that you do not cloud the issue with extraneous information.

Think of a practice or procedure, referred to here as 'Procedure X', that has been established for some time, the value of which you have cause to question.

Assessing and planning

In this part of the process, set up the premises for rational thinking by making an initial assessment of the problem and by planning for the development of an argument.

- What is Procedure X?
- Why is Procedure X done?

- How is Procedure X done?
- When is Procedure X done?
- What are the outcomes of Procedure X?
- Why do you believe that Procedure X is of questionable value?
- How do you propose to amend Procedure X?

From your responses to the previous questions, state the problem, giving a preliminary hypothesis about the expected relationships between the variables you have identified. If you are unable to state a hypothesis at this point you may need to spend more time assessing the problem, and you may need to collect more facts related to Procedure X.

- What words and language are associated commonly with Procedure X?
- Why are certain words and language associated commonly with Procedure X?
- Is there any evidence of misuse of words and language in Procedure X?
- Could the words and language associated commonly with Procedure X be stated differently?
- What healthcare problems are associated with Procedure X?

Implementing

In this part of the process, develop an argument by analysing the issues and assumptions operating in the situation.

- What arguments are made to support the continuation of Procedure X in its present form?
- What healthcare assumptions underlie the support of Procedure X in its present form?
- What premises support the argument for Procedure X in its present form?
- Do these premises follow logically to provide sound conclusions?
- If not, why not?
- What inferences have been made and in what ways are they plausible in supporting Procedure X in its present form?

Now is the time to formulate and clarify your own beliefs about Procedure X as stated in your hypothesis.

- What arguments are made to support the discontinuation of Procedure X in its present form?
- What healthcare assumptions underlie the opposition to Procedure X in its present form?

- On what premises are these arguments for opposing Procedure X in its present form based?
- Do these premises follow logically to provide sound conclusions?
- If not, why not?
- What inferences have been made and in what ways are they plausible in opposing Procedure X in its present form?

To test the consequences of the position that Procedure X is of questionable value in its present form, you need to implement some changes, or 'apply the findings' of rational deliberation in the practices associated with Procedure X. The changes would need to be based on the results of rational discussion and decision-making, but they might include factors such as the time of day, the frequency of the procedure, preparations for Procedure X, the sequence of the method and activities following Procedure X.

Evaluating

In this part of the process, you review the problem in the light of all the information gained through the process of technical reflection.

- What information has been gained to date through implementing the technical reflection process?
- In what ways can you verify, corroborate and justify claims, beliefs, conclusions, decisions and actions taken in this process?
- What are the reasons for your beliefs and conclusions regarding this issue?
- What are your value judgements about this issue?
- To what extent can you claim that the conclusions you have reached are sound?
- What other possible consequences may transpire due to the conclusions reached by this process?

Make a succinct statement to either confirm or disconfirm the hypothesis as stated at the outset of this process.

You have just been through the technical reflection process to generate empirical knowledge, to amend and improve a clinical procedure. Congratulations!

An example of technical reflection

If you lost your way in the previous section, or found parts of the process difficult to follow, this section provides an example of technical reflection to assist you. The example responds to questions listed in the technical reflection process above.

A group of midwives working in a neonatal intensive care unit were concerned about whether frequent handling of neonates for procedures was resulting in the babies developing hypothermia. They knew that compromised neonates have difficulty in maintaining their body temperature because of factors associated with prematurity and low birth weight, and they also knew that parental touch is important for bonding and comfort for neonates requiring intensive care. The midwives decided to undertake an investigation as part of their routine care of the neonates focusing on the effects of handling by noting temperature changes in the neonates. Their observations over a 48-hour period showed that neonates' body temperatures fluctuated and decreased in relation to procedural handling. To demonstrate the hypothermic effect of frequent handling for procedures and to gain their colleagues' cooperation in reducing unnecessary handling, the midwives decided to present a sound argument at the interdisciplinary meeting that handling of the neonates resulted in fluctuations and decreased neonatal temperature recordings and that procedural handling needed to be restricted in favour of parental touch.

This example shows how the midwives used technical reflection to present a sound argument to the interdisciplinary committee.

Assessing and planning

In this part of the process, set up the premises for rational thinking by making an initial assessment of the problem and planning for the development of an argument.

- **What is Procedure X?** The procedure/questionable practice is frequent procedural handling of neonates receiving intensive care.
- **Why is Procedure X done?** To ensure that neonates are monitored carefully, so all their needs are met.
- **How is Procedure X done?** Neonates are handled for procedures in relation to the observation of their physiological status, and their treatment, feeding and hygiene needs.
- **When is Procedure X done?** Neonatal procedural handling occurs at least every 30 minutes, sometimes more frequently.
- **What are the outcomes of Procedure X?** The neonates are monitored frequently and carefully and their physiological needs are met.
- **Why do you believe that Procedure X is of questionable value?** Frequent procedural handling of neonates is of questionable value because it results in body temperature fluctuations and hypothermia.
- **How do you propose to amend Procedure X?** The proposed amendment is to restrict neonatal procedural handling to two-hourly, by grouping procedures and favouring parental touch at set times.

From your responses to the previous questions, state the problem, giving a preliminary hypothesis about the expected relationships between the variables you have identified. If you are unable to state a hypothesis at this point you may need to spend more time assessing the problem, and you may need to collect more facts related to Procedure X (the practice of frequent procedural handling of neonates is questionable, because it results in neonatal body temperature fluctuations and hypothermia).

- **What words and language are associated commonly with Procedure X?** The words and language associated with frequent procedural handling of neonates are: 'How is Baby B doing?' 'What are the obs?' 'Is a feeding due?' 'What is Baby C's urinary output?'
- **Why are certain words and language associated commonly with Procedure X?** The words and language associated with frequent procedural handling are related directly to assessing and meeting the neonates' physiological, dietary and hygiene needs.
- **Is there any evidence of misuse of words and language in Procedure X?** The 'misuse' of words and language is minimal, in that they reflect a focus on meeting the neonates' needs, but the emphasis is on procedural touch, not on facilitating parental touch and minimizing neonatal handling overall.
- **Could the words and language associated commonly with Procedure X be stated differently?** Yes, if the interdisciplinary team members look at the ways they communicate about neonatal procedures, they will identify their tendency to focus on their need to undertake frequent procedures, in preference to parental touch. For example, differently stated the sentences could be: 'We need to attend to neonates' needs, in relation to grouping activities', 'Baby B's mother is coming to the unit at 10 a.m. We know Baby B is doing fine. Let's leave the obs and other procedures until Baby B's mother arrives'.
- **What healthcare problems are associated with Procedure X?** Frequent procedural handling of neonates ensures that neonatal needs are met, but it intensifies the likelihood of neonatal temperature fluctuations and hypothermia.

Implementing

In this part of the process, develop an argument by analysing the issues and assumptions operating in the situation.

- **What arguments are made to support the continuation of Procedure X in its present form?** Interdisciplinary team members who support the continuation of frequent procedural handling of neonates at least every

30 minutes argue that physiological dysfunction happens rapidly in pre-term and low birth weight babies and that frequent monitoring is necessary to detect any deterioration.

- **What health care assumptions underlie the support of Procedure X in its present form?** That all neonates, regardless of apparent physiological indicators of good health status, need to be handled frequently for procedures. Assumptions may also be that interdisciplinary team members will have less anxiety about neonates' progress if they can be assured by frequent procedural handling that babies' health indicators are within normal limits. There may also be an implicit assumption that if neonates are to be handled, the best use of touch is for procedures, not parental contact.

- **What premises support the argument for Procedure X in its present form?** The premises are as stated previously: neonates will be monitored frequently, so their needs can be met.

- **Do these premises follow logically to provide sound conclusions? If not, why not?** No, because the interdisciplinary team members' assumptions have not been made explicit. In addition, the premises do not take the hypothermic effects of frequent procedural handling into account, nor is there any consideration of the neonates' needs for parental touch.

- **What inferences have been made and in what ways are they plausible in supporting Procedure X in its present form?** The inference is that if neonates are handled at least every 30 minutes then their physiological indicators can be monitored and their needs can be met immediately. This inference is plausible in the sense that neonates require observation, but it is not plausible in specifying every 30 minutes, as it does not necessarily follow that neonates require that time frame for the most efficient outcomes, nor does it take into account the resultant hypothermic effects and the preference for procedural touch over parental touch.

Now is the time to formulate and clarify your own beliefs about Procedure X as stated in your hypothesis.

- **What arguments are made to support the discontinuation of Procedure X in its present form?** That although neonates require procedural touch, this does not have to be frequent, at intervals of 30 minutes, because overhandling results in neonatal temperature fluctuations and hypothermia, as shown by a documented 48 hour investigation in the neonatal intensive care unit.

- **What healthcare assumptions underlie the opposition to Procedure X in its present form?** Assumptions opposing the procedure of frequent procedural touch are that neonates' physiological indicators can be observed through non-touch means and that grouping of procedures by interdisciplinary team members will minimize neonatal handling and favour parental touch, thus reducing the likelihood of hypothermic effects of overhandling. The previously unexpressed assumptions are also challenged that interdisciplinary team members who continue the frequent neonatal handling are actually using it to minimize their own anxieties and to preference procedural touch over parental touch.

- **On what premises are these arguments for opposing Procedure X in its present form based?** That neonates require procedures, but the present tendency to handle neonates at least very 30 minutes is resulting in temperature fluctuations and hypothermia. Also, as neonatal touch is to be limited, it is best reserved, where possible, for parental contact.
- **Do these premises follow logically to provide sound conclusions? If not, why not?** Yes.
- **What inferences have been made and in what ways are they plausible in opposing Procedure X in its present form?** One inference is that if neonatal handling is limited then the neonates' needs will be met without hypothermic effects. Another series of connected inferences is that if the procedural touch is grouped into two hourly intervals or less, where possible, then more non-touch continuous means of monitoring can be used and essential procedural touch can be combined with regular parental contact.

To test the consequences of the position that Procedure X is of questionable value in its present form, you need to implement some changes, or 'apply the findings' of rational deliberation in the practices associated with Procedure X. The changes would need to be based on the results of rational discussion and decision-making, but they might include factors such as the time of day, the frequency of the procedure, preparations for Procedure X, the sequence of the method and activities following Procedure X.

Evaluating

In this part of the process, you review the problem in the light of all the information gained through the process of technical reflection. We will assume that the midwives' sound argument was successful at the interdisciplinary meeting, and frequent procedural touching of neonates has been discontinued in favour of grouping care activities every two hours or less, combined with parental contact and increased means of non-touch neonatal monitoring devices.

- **What information has been gained to date through implementing the technical reflection process?** Although it took some time to assure all the members of the interdisciplinary team, the majority of the healthcare professionals have noticed that the parents are happy with the amended procedure. Even more importantly, there have been less fluctuations in neonatal body temperatures and hypothermia, and associated physiological indicators such as neonatal blood glucose levels have been more stable.

- **In what ways can you verify, corroborate and justify claims, beliefs, conclusions, decisions and actions taken in this process?** The amended procedure has resulted in less disruption to neonates, allowing them to rest for longer periods. Parents have expressed delight at being able to touch their baby more often and to be more involved in witnessing their care. Physiological indicators, such as more stable neonatal temperatures and blood glucose levels have been connected directly to the reduction of procedural touch.

- **What are the reasons for your beliefs and conclusions regarding this issue?** The issue of frequent procedural handling of neonates has been related to the often unexpressed need of healthcare members to attend to their work, to assure themselves of the neonates' progress. For example, there was limited communication in the interdisciplinary team about the tendency to disturb neonates frequently and scant attention had been paid to considering the amount of handling overall. After a period of grouping care activities, the direct connection between frequent procedural touch and hypothermia demonstrated the need to reduce overall touch and to favour parental touch wherever possible.

- **What are your value judgements about this issue?** That parents have the right to be involved in their baby's care and to bond with their child as soon as possible. Interdisciplinary team members involved in neonatal intensive care should meet the changing physiological needs of the neonate and keep the family's needs to touch and bond with their child central to their practice.

- **To what extent can you claim that the conclusions you have reached are sound?** The conclusions are sound, in that the amended procedure has resulted in greater benefits to neonates, parents and healthcare professionals, because it fulfils the neonates' physiological needs for temperature control, the parents' needs for touch and bonding, and the interdisciplinary team members' needs to meet the needs of neonates requiring intensive care.

- **What other possible consequences may transpire due to the conclusions reached by this process?** That other unexamined neonatal intensive care procedures and routines may be questioned and changed through a technical reflection process and research projects, where required.

- **Make a succinct statement to either confirm or disconfirm the hypothesis as stated at the outset of this process.** The hypothesis is confirmed that the frequent procedural touch results in neonatal temperature fluctuations and hypothermia and needs to be discontinued, because neonates' physiological needs can be met by grouping of procedures into two-hourly intervals, where possible, in conjunction with non-touch neonatal monitoring devices and regular parental touch.

Author's reflection

I began nurse training in 1968 in Tasmania, a small island state, south of the mainland of Australia. Our group introduced the new nurses' uniform, which was a light-coloured garment with no starch, unlike the Florence Nightingale original design worn by my seniors, but we retained the stripes on our bonnets to denote our lowly level in the nursing hierarchy. My training was just that – training – like any person receives who needs to keep in lockstep with a sponsoring organization involved in high-risk activities intending to keep its good reputation, such as a police department, an army or a hospital.

Empirical knowledge and technical skills were of the highest importance in my nurse training, because they were the mark of a 'real nurse'. My training ensured that I internalized the technicalities of nursing, so that I would be safe to practise. I was 17 years old, so I was grateful for the training, as it safeguarded me and the people for whom I cared, until I was mature enough to think independently, to synthesize the knowledge I took in initially by rote learning. For example, I remember one of the tutor sisters writing definitions on a blackboard and every Monday in Preliminary Training School (PTS) we were tested on them, and expected to remember every word in the exact order. For example, a mantra which has been embedded in my brain ever since is: 'Melaena is a black, sticky, tarry, offensive stool, due to blood which has undergone changes in the alimentary canal'.

The clinical procedures were also learned by rote, for example, ten steps for bed-making and a precise order for undertaking sterile dressings. No lateral thinking was required or encouraged, rather, there were strict rules for technical skills, for example, 'when pouring medications from bottles on the drug trolley, the label must be held in the palm of the hand'. This rule was not explained, but I imagine the precaution was to prevent the label from becoming messy and obscured. For years after PTS I applied this rule to all other bottles, such as sauce and wine, even though it was an irrational practice, until I eventually turned it into a joke and desisted. I wonder how many obsessive-compulsive disorders are created and nurtured in training camps and schools?

The unquestioning indoctrination of my nurse training meant I was subjected to many outmoded nursing practices. For example, I often 'ran myself ragged' trying to keep track of far too many fluid balance charts and in taking frequent routine postoperative observations on patients who had long since recovered well from anaesthesia. It took me a while to summon the courage to question pointless orders, which served mainly to perpetuate my subservience, keep me busy and to give me a great deal of personal conflict when I could not keep up with the pace and weight of the workload.

When I look back now, I smile to think of myself as 'Nurse Bugg – Nurse Efficiency!' I was so very serious as a nurse in training and most of the time I was in a state of high anxiety. I guess this was a good thing as it kept me from becoming too big-headed and my wholehearted intention to do things properly and on time meant that I won the hospital's bedside nursing prize and did no harm to the people in my care. The regimentation of my nurse training gave me rock solid clinical skills and there was no doubt that after three years of repetition I had sure and solid mastery of a wide range of proficiencies. It is regrettable, though, that much of the knowledge and many of the clinical procedures could have been internalized better through a system of experiential learning, critical thinking and reflection, rather than rote learning and the sheer terror of making a mistake as a junior nurse.

Summary

Questions about clinical procedures can be answered quickly and effectively through technical reflection. This chapter reviewed some previous information given in this book, connected directly to technical reflection, explaining some of the reasons why technical reflection is used for specific purposes and why it creates practical answers to clinical problems. The relationships were reviewed between empirical knowledge and the scientific method, and how the process for technical reflection fits with these ideas. The connections were described between technical reflection and evidence-based practice and it was suggested that the two processes are highly complementary.

Technical reflection is based on a form of empirical knowledge generation, which is useful for clinical practice. Technical reflection as an amalgam of Bandman and Bandman's (1995) view of scientific reasoning and the functions of critical thinkers, the features of critical thinking and thinkers described by van Hooft *et al.* (1995) and the problem-solving steps of the nursing process (Wilkinson 1996). The chapter provided an example of technical reflection so you can see how the process can be applied to clinical procedures and policies in your work.

Key points

- Questions about outmoded clinical procedures and policies can be answered through technical reflection.

- For healthcare professionals, technical interest is associated with task-related competence, such as clinical procedures; therefore technical reflection involves empirical knowledge, rationality, the scientific method, critical thinking and problem-solving.
- The evidence-based movement in healthcare professions is testing the validity of long-standing procedures and is seeking to replace old untested and unproven approaches with newer research-based ones.
- 'Assessing and planning' is the part of the technical reflection process in which you set up the premises for rational thinking by making an initial assessment of the problem and planning for the development of an argument.
- 'Implementing' is the part of the process in which you develop an argument by analysing the issues and assumptions operating in the situation.
- 'Evaluating' is the part of the process in which you review the problem in the light of all the information gained through the process of technical reflection.
- The outcomes of technical reflection can be immediate, if the process has been shared with, and the findings endorsed by, the key people who are in a position to influence and ratify healthcare practice.
- In whatever situations you use it, technical reflection has the potential for allowing you to think critically and to reason scientifically, so that you can critique and adapt present procedures to better ones as necessary. You may also be able to predict likely outcomes for similar procedures and improve many work practices through objective and systematic lines of inquiry.

5   Practical reflection

Introduction

This chapter reviews some information connected directly to practical reflection, before guiding you through the practical reflection process and giving examples of how practical reflection can be used by healthcare professionals.

When I turned my attention towards practical reflection, I realized that this would involve an adjustment of what has been used previously in the work of Smyth (1986a, 1986b) and Street (1991), with an adaptation to emphasize the communicative nature of this type of reflection. Therefore, practical reflection retains some of the questions used previously within the process of experiencing, interpreting and learning. Experiencing involves retelling a practice story so that you experience it again in as much detail as possible. Interpreting involves clarifying and explaining the meaning of a communicative action situation. Learning involves creating new insights and integrating them into your existing awareness and knowledge.

Practical reflection is important in itself. The reason for this is that there is immense value in reflecting for the purposes of interpreting and learning from work life. Although change may not be an explicit aim of practical reflection, it is still possible, through new insights that follow from raised awareness. However, while practical reflection is helpful, it has limitations in what it can offer you. Through the medium of language, practical reflection will help you to understand the interpersonal basis of human experiences and will also offer you the potential for creating new knowledge which interprets the meaning of your lived experience, context and subjectivity. You can experience changes through practical reflection, although that is not its primary aim. The changes will be based on your raised awareness of the nature and effects of a wide range of communicative matters pertaining to your practice.

However, practical reflection will not offer you the objective means to observe and analyse work procedures through a scientific method, because it does not have an interest in instrumental action. Also, practical reflection will not give you a process for making a radical critique of the constraining forces and power influences within your work settings. The reason for this is that, although practical reflection can raise awareness through insights into communicative action, unlike emancipatory reflection it does not have transformative action as its primary concern.

Review of previous ideas

In Chapter 3 I described practical reflection in relation to interpretive knowledge and practical interests. Practical reflection is related to interpretive knowledge, because it centres on people and values their perceptions of their life experiences and their ability to communicate them. People communicate through language, symbols, ceremonies, rituals, art forms and other behavioural practices. Of all the means of communication, the main way of making and sharing meaning is through speaking words that convey ideas, concepts, theories, propositions and so on. One of the most important reasons for language and interpersonal discussion is the communication of human experience, because people assign significance to what is happening within their own bodies and lives, and to similar concerns of other people. Practical reflection focuses on human experience and communication to make sense out of these phenomena through experiencing, interpreting and learning from them.

Interpretive knowledge centres on people, because of their perceptions of their life experiences and their ability to communicate them. The underlying concepts of interpretive knowledge include interpersonal understanding through attention to people's lived experience, context and subjectivity.

Lived experience means knowing what it is like to live a life in a particular time, place and set of circumstances. It involves the interpretation of experiences, which make up the fabric of human existence, once they have been opened up to reflection. It is only through reflection that people can make sense of their lived experiences, because time must elapse – whether it is moments or years – to sort through the meaning of experiences. Daily life is always moving forward towards the next experience and it is so easy to get caught up in it and to just let it happen. If you think of what it is like to be a human, the movement forward of life is within a body in a social world, and in respect to everything which occurs as part of living. In a sense, we are propelled forward by the prospect of tomorrow, and we cannot help but accumulate experiences along the way. This being so, there is a need to make sense of lived experience, in order to prepare for further forward movement by reflecting on what has happened, why and how, so that we can learn in the present and project these new insights into the future. Therefore, lived experience is an important concept in understanding interpretive knowledge and how it fits into practical reflection.

Context means all of the features of the time and place in which people find themselves, in which they locate their lives. If you think now of your context, how would you describe it? My context presently is that I am living on the far north coast of New South Wales, Australia. This is where I do honorary work as an emeritus professor and where I reside with my partner Chris and son Michael. My context is also described by my age, gender and social and political affiliations, such as my friends, colleagues and other relationships and my work and home interests. I could go on to describe more and more of my context and the more I describe, the broader and deeper my context would become. I cannot help but be connected to my context in all of its features, because I relate to it as part of myself and, in turn, it tells me who I am. Interpretive knowledge is explained in part by context, because it situates people in their experiences and gives them some markers for making sense of their lives. This is also how it relates to practical reflection.

Subjectivity refers to the individual's sensing of inner and external events, which includes personal experiences and truths that may or may not be like other people's subjective experiences and truths. In this book I am using the word 'subjectivity' in an uncomplicated way, which avoids the philosophical arguments differentiating it from objectivity. In relation to interpretive knowledge, subjectivity is the means through which individuals sense phenomena inside and outside themselves. Therefore, it is a form of knowledge within the person as subject – that is, the person who relates towards objects of attention. Subjectivity is a part of interpretive knowledge, because the person as the knower, who makes sense of his or her experiences, creates it.

Intersubjectivity refers to how individuals take account of one another in the social world to make sense of their experiences. We tend to live in social circumstances and therefore we need to take account of other people and their experiences. Interpretive knowledge is formed in part by people in dialogue with one another, negotiating the sense they make out of experiences by sharing and contesting meaning in human communication.

In summary, interpretive knowledge emerges from the perspectives of people engaged actively in their lives and it includes and values what people feel and think. Judgements as to the usefulness and 'truthfulness' of the accounts are based on the relative indicators, such as the nature of lived experience, context and subjectivity.

In Chapter 3 I also introduced the idea of practical interest, derived from the work of Jurgen Habermas. To some extent, I have already linked practical interest and interpretive knowledge, but you may find further explanation useful at this point. Practical interest involves human interaction or 'communicative action', which involves reciprocal expectations about behaviour, which are defined and understood by the people involved. In other words, and put into the negative, if it did not exist, we would have no means of making sense of communication if we did not agree on what certain words and symbols mean. Through this lack of consensus, it follows that we would not have a common basis for agreeing on the relevant action needed in certain circumstances.

In a work setting, communicative action translates to something as familiar as the communication patterns that are set up by clinicians and the people with whom they come into contact. Communicative action in healthcare professions relates to agreeing on and acting upon shared communication norms and expectations. Social norms, or sets of expectations for behaviour, are created over time by people who are in consensus about what is expected in certain situations. The social norms are enforced through sanctions, which ensure that people recognize and honour their responsibilities in the reciprocal behaviour. Thus communicative action is a rich source of interest for practical reflection. As the main intentions of practical interests are to describe and explain human interaction, they are concerned with interpretation and explanation through practical reflection, which in turn creates interpretive knowledge.

Reflector

When you are next at work, watch what happens when people are speaking with one another. Do certain combinations of people relate in a 'typical' fashion (e.g. nurse with physiotherapist, social worker with doctor, occupational therapist with relative, speech therapist with patient and so on)? Are there any noticeable patterns in the ways healthcare professionals relate to people in authority, as opposed to people at their occupational level or below in the work setting hierarchy?

Practice story

Ruth is in her late fifties and she has been practising as an occupational therapist for 35 years. Ruth worked initially in a rehabilitation unit for a couple of years, then stopped to raise a family, before going back to work in mental health. In the last 22 years Ruth has been working in community health and hospitals in part-time and full-time positions. Her work has involved facilitating clients being rehabilitated from mental health facilities into group homes in the community and she has managed group homes and the daily functioning of the residents. Using the practical reflection process, Ruth related a story involving difficulties in communication at work.

There is an ongoing client, whose care I had for years. This client had multiple disabilities – cerebral palsy, ageing (he was 65) and he was totally blind. He was cared for by an even older, ageing mother, who did not go as far as litigation, but she certainly made many ministerial complaints. I was involved in one complaint with the mother. The mother uses the system as best she can. She has looked after her son, took him out of a nursing home when he was 22 and now he is 65. He is her only child and so she is entitled to everything she can get. They are on pensions and they do not have any other assets whatsoever, just the pensions. He has a blind pension; she now has an aged pension. She is between 85 and 90 and still living with her son and professional carers come in.

At times, in which I was involved, she was not happy with the care, frequently sacked the carers, wore out a couple – at least one physio, a couple of occupational therapists – and the case came to me. The reason it came to me (I was the last one there) is because I am also senior in years, and I have lots of experience and very grey hair. I was close to the client's age and this has been a benefit. So, this lady was very difficult. Strategies were in place – it was difficult before I got there – but I have been involved with her and her son on and off for over 16 years. The mother had given her son so much care and I respect that and I have come to respect her role as a mother as well, and that's what helped in the final outcome, I think.

But, there were difficulties always. I would prescribe a wheelchair, several times over the years – about each five years the wheelchair would need replacing. The successive wheelchairs were never as good as the initial one she had. We tried to order an exact copy, but in the mother's view, no wheelchair was as good as the first, which became 'not available'. We got the closest model to the first, but it was not good enough, as she had faith in the first model. It was hard for her to appreciate that her son was much younger then, he was a lot fitter, he could actually walk a tiny distance in those days, making a stand transfer much safer. It was difficult for her to understand that he was ageing at a faster rate than she, because his cerebral palsy affected three limbs and he was blind. Fortunately, he could hear very well, and he could follow instructions very well and he'd adapted to his blindness. He wasn't blind from birth so he could understand visual instructions. He had sight until he was 21 – one eye went at 11 and the other at 21. It took a lot of pleasure out of his life. He was a little bit 'DD' [developmentally disabled] as well, but he can speak, even though it is difficult to understand his speech. But his mother looked after him.

He has a normal diet, which was good. And, he was very big, very tall, and he was gradually putting on weight, so transfers were increasingly difficult, so the chair was blamed. So, eventually, we changed the chair, we got another brand, brand number three, and ultimately that was rejected, and we went to brand number four, and then five. Brand number four worked for some time, that was accepted – never as good – but accepted.

Other players involved were a little bit of social work, also management had to be involved, because of the complaints. The wheelchair was only one issue – there were other complaints of community aged carers' lack of ability to care. Carers were trained and paid to care for him. The social worker got involved in selecting a suitable care agency, which burnt out eventually, then another agency was selected, and as far as I know that agency is going fine.

Critical friend response

Critical friend: *Getting back to you and your part in this story, it sounds to me like you did everything you could.*

Ruth: *I did everything I could that I knew of at the time, but maybe if we had better suppliers, or maybe if I had contracted a supplier in a capital city, and got the department to pay for the freight, we may have been able to trial wheelchairs.*

Critical friend: *So, the ongoing saga of the chair created a focus that was an ongoing frustration for you.*

Ruth: *Oh, definitely, for me and many clinicians. I wasn't the only one. And another frustration is, that we got to the last chair I prescribed for this fellow and it was generally accepted, even though there were a couple of complaints about the chair itself – it was a little but flimsy and adaptations had to be made at the manufacturer's expense, and that was resolved. Then management became involved, saying: 'We know the history of this person, we'd better get another opinion in'. So, I wasn't happy with that. Someone came in over me and got another occupational therapist in.*

Critical friend: *The implication being . . .*

Ruth: *. . . that I am not adequate. I didn't really feel that I was inadequate, and I could see the value of what management were saying, because of the long history with the client.*

Practice story

Ruth went on to explain that the contracted occupational therapist recommended a couple of changes, and Ruth remembered thinking: 'I've known him 15 years and you've only met him once or twice.' Ruth acknowledged that the occupational therapist did an excellent job and the recommendations for changes could have worked, but when she did a follow-up after that, the mother carer said: 'Why did they do that? Why didn't they accept what you said?' Ruth said that when the mother carer came in to defend her, she was 'gobsmacked'. The mother carer, the client and Ruth privately agreed not to change the wheelchair. Ruth realized that there was a change in trust between them after 10 to 12 years of interacting. A bond was created between them and the mother made no complaints about Ruth after that, and over the years she became quite supportive. Ruth explained that because of the potential for things to 'blow up' with mother and staff, when any decision was made they wrote a contract and she had to sign it. Ruth was uncomfortable with it but she said nothing to the mother initially. When the mother also became uncomfortable and refused to sign contracts, they tended to agree and negotiated care on trust.

Ruth's hopes for the practice outcomes related to the wheelchair prescription, to make a safer outcome for the carer, the client, or both, and to have a wheelchair to continue to meet his needs, given his disabilities and growing obesity. Ruth's hopes were related to her ideals about providing for what suits the client, not herself as the technical provider. Ruth concluded: 'Each client is so different, and even though there are uniform diagnoses, there's no uniform prescription.'

Ruth described the sources of the way she communicates, including church fellowship, and growing up with a very deaf, ageing grandfather. For over 35 years Ruth has worked with a range of people, mostly aged, so growing up with an aged grandfather provided a vocabulary to use with an aged person. She speaks differently to clients, by speaking slower, louder, clearly and sometimes a little simpler. Ruth's mother also made her speak very clearly and she was insistent on very good grammar and encouraged Ruth in receiving a tertiary education. Ruth also identified other communication sources such as being involved in the community, playing sports and communicating with people her own age and younger. She is married to a tradesman, so she can talk a manual type of vocabulary. When she reflected on the sources, she realized that trust is important for her and the way she communicates.

I was taught to establish a rapport firstly, and I've always done that. I will go into a home and I will talk about them or the photo on the wall, or the plant at the front door. I'll find something in common to communicate about, to establish a rapport and where I am coming from. I try to give a little bit of myself, like: 'I like that plant, because . . .' or: 'Oh, I know that person in that photo'. I try to establish a common link first, so they know something about me. Part of the self-disclosure I use, I was taught never to do, but I have found that it works. It builds trust because they get to know a little about me, because they are going to reveal a lot about themselves and I am in their personal space. I feel they have a right to know a bit about me, to establish that rapport and trust and I will always do that before I do an assessment of whatever it is. The rapport with the mother carer was slow, because of her defences, but I think I did ultimately achieve my goals, in a 15-year process. Initially, I was seen as a much younger person, maybe a threat.

Some of us would like to deal with a client alone, and the mother often prevented that, so a rapport had to be established with the mother. I was 'on edge' a lot. I was apprehensive a lot, so I had to be brief and direct in my communication with this client. 'What's the need? Show me.' We defined the problem and had to be in a three-way agreement and list the problems if they were multiple. We had to be very definite in our communication, so my communication was more minimal than any other client and I tried to give the client some 'one to one' wherever possible. He was denied that, often, in the earlier stages, not so much in the later stages as the mother built up trust, she would leave the room. But, she is a mother and wants to defend the rights of her son and wants the best outcome and I always respected that.

We did have agreed hopes, but I also knew we could not achieve the perfect outcomes the mother was demanding – the perfect wheelchair did not exist, the perfect bath did not exist, the perfect toilet transfer did not exist. We could not restore that son's abilities, or rather the abilities he never had and that was an ongoing problem.

Unfortunately, there weren't many rewards in this case. The penalties were ministerial complaints over and over in the earlier years. I was named in one of them, I think it may have been about a cushion, but I was not cited in any written complaints. The complaints were continuous about carers, and all those who set foot inside the front door – nobody was perfect – so it had to be assumed, unfortunately, that there could be a phone call or ministerial complaint, which is regrettable. However, as the years progressed the complaints didn't come to me, about me, but I always expected it, unfortunately. Complaints would come for others, the focus would shift from caregiver to caregiver and we were just waiting for when it was our turn. Was it the physio's turn, was it the dietician's turn, was it the occupational therapist's turn?

Eventually, the rewards came for me personally when she accepted: 'Yes, this piece of equipment does work.'

When I come to a complex client, who has a complex medical condition, environmental needs and equipment needs, there is lot to bring together for the best outcome. So, I sometimes doubt my ability, and need to bounce off other clinicians. I definitely need the support. I came through this without needing others particularly, to come in and be involved, but I found support in the technical advisers of equipment – they were very good. Personality wise, I would bounce off other clinicians. I would debrief with other clinicians.

Re. expectations of others – don't expect a perfect outcome – never – because no human being is perfect. All the clients we see have disabilities that are reported to us, but there is always something else when we get there and there are personalities and histories – always more to people than we expect. To expect a perfect outcome is too high. Define the problem and try to get an agreement on the best outcome, and a variety of options.

I have learned to go slowly and I definitely define the problem and trial equipment. I learned to trial equipment much better – not to assume, like, if someone gave me a diagnosis, not to assume, 'Well, I'll need this and this and this' – it is not always the case, I've learnt that, the hard way. This practice experience made me change a little bit – not be so swift with interactions and assessments – I would have liked to be a bit quicker with them, but I've learnt I can't do that with aged people. It's taught me to look at the problems in more detail than even before. I've learnt to not assume. I once assumed a lot more. To follow up whenever there's doubt. 'Is it working for you?' I didn't follow up so well, but this taught me to follow up the controversial clients, in cases where equipment may go wrong. They need a follow-up phone call: 'Is this working for you?'

The process of practical reflection

At this point, you may find it helpful to refer to Chapter 2, in which I suggested some prerequisites for reflecting. There are many strategies for reflecting, which you can use alone or in combination. If you have been reading through this book sequentially, by now you will be equipped with some of the literature which affirms the usefulness of reflective practice and some stories from other healthcare professionals who have begun reflecting on their practice. You may also have undertaken a 'warm up' exercise, in which I encouraged you to think about the person and professional you are now in the light of childhood memories and rules for living. In the previous chapter, you may have also applied technical reflective processes to procedural work requiring improvement through rational processes. We are now at the point at which it is time to reflect on some practice incidents, which could benefit from practical reflection.

The focus of your stories is you, so that you can gain new insights from your experiences. In the exercise that follows, you will reflect on your own work setting and practice, because these stories require you to be active and central to what is happening. You can use the process as a means of exploring any questions and concerns related to the interpersonal basis of your work experiences. When you have recorded one scenario, you can go on to reflect on as many as you choose. Although a daily reflective habit is excellent, if you can manage only one focused attempt each week that will be useful. You might find that your reflection is more a matter of quality than quantity. As I explained previously, it is important to keep a compilation of all your reflections, because you will need them to compare your insights over time. They will show you your main issues and how you are working through them using reflective processes.

In considering these questions, you are making an interpretation of human interactions in your practice. You will begin to see that, even though you are often at the centre of the action, you are certainly not the only person contributing to the situation. Human communication is complex and by looking at the relationships and shared norms you will raise your awareness about your own values and actions, and how they relate to those held and done by other people. This means that you will have a greater understanding of your own communication patterns and those of the people with whom you work.

Think of an incident at work in which you were undertaking your usual work activities involving interpersonal communication, that you felt did not go well. In other words, the situation did not develop the positive outcomes you had envisioned. Record your responses by whatever means you prefer, ensuring that you can review your answers for later analysis.

Experiencing

Experiencing involves retelling a practice story so that you experience it again in as much detail as possible.

In this part of the process, it is important to recall the sights, sounds, smells, people and any other features which had a bearing on the incident. It might help if you shut your eyes and take yourself back in your imagination to that time. Alternatively, you might like to begin the process by getting ready emotionally through creative means, such as by playing music, painting or any of the other strategies mentioned in Chapter 2.

When you have a clear image of the situation, write down or represent creatively a full description of the experience. Refer to yourself in the first person, so that you remain engaged centrally and actively in the story. Let your thinking flow so that you portray your head image as faithfully as possible. Respond to the following questions to build up a 'thick description' of the experience:

- What was happening?
- When was it happening?
- Where was it happening?
- Why was it happening?
- Who was involved?
- How were you involved?
- What was the setting like, in terms of its smells, sounds and sights?
- What were the outcomes of the situation?
- How did you feel honestly about the situation?

Let the reflection end when it exhausts itself, then review what you have written or represented in some other creative form. Compare the image in your head with your representation of the event. How do the image and the representation of the reflection compare? If the words or other means of creative expression do not do justice to your head image, go back and elaborate further to ensure that you have encapsulated the experience as well as you possibly can.

Interpreting

Interpreting involves clarifying and explaining the meaning of a situation in which communication led to action.

You should have before you a fully descriptive scenario of the situational and communicative aspects of your experience. To make sense of the story, you will need to revisit the account to locate yourself and the communication patterns that were set up with the other people. To find the communicative action features in the story, read the account or review the creative representation and ask yourself:

- What were my hopes for the practice outcomes in this story?
- How were my hopes related to my ideals of what constitutes 'good' practice?
- What are the sources in my life and work for my ideas and values for communicative aspects of my practice?
- In what ways do I embody them now in the way I communicate at work?
- What was my communicative role in this situation?
- To what extent did I achieve my communicative role?
- How did my interpretation of my role affect my relations with the people in the situation?

- What are the shared communication norms and expectations in this situation? In other words, how did everyone else in the story interpret their roles and what did they seem to expect in the situation?
- To what extent were social norms, or sets of expectations for behaviour, operating in this situation?
- What system of spoken and unspoken rewards and penalties was in place to maintain and control socially accepted behaviours in this situation?
- Were the usual communicative norms and sanctions altered in this situation?

Learning

Learning involves creating new insights and integrating them into your existing awareness and knowledge.

- What does this scenario tell me about my expectations of myself?
- What does this scenario tell me about my expectations of other people?
- What have I learned from this situation?
- What kinds of adaptations are possible in my work relationships?
- How do I fit these new insights into my present ways of regarding communicative action in my work?

Record your responses to these questions and discuss them with a critical friend. When you are ready, apply your new learning to your work situation.

An example of practical reflection

Christine is a social worker, aged 'about 50', who has been working since she was 23, in a range of positions. Christine has been a reflective practitioner from training days using reflective processes in a variety of ways, but since the year 2000 the best source of reflection for her has been through narrative therapy, which contextualizes people in their whole life stories.

Experiencing

Experiencing involves retelling a practice story so that you experience it again in as much detail as possible.

- **What? When? Where? Why? Who? How were you involved? What was the setting like?** This is a practice story in which I engaged in some reflective practice with someone. One of my responsibilities has been clinically supervising other people and that goes really well if there is a resonance between you, but it can be much more challenging. Supervision can be with other social workers, but it can also be with people from other disciplines. Supervision can be clinical or administrative and it can be case management, or any of those things. There was one instance where this particular worker and I come from really different life experience, I think, and what I was aware of in our interactions was a growing situation where certain comments that would be made by the worker would kind of press my buttons. Then, rather than being able to stay in a grounded, centred space, which is where you need to be when you are providing supervision, I would find myself becoming reactive.

- **What were the outcomes of the situation?** As a consequence, on one particular occasion that I can think of, I remember saying something to that worker that wasn't helpful, and certainly wasn't helpful in terms of the purpose for our meeting.

- **How did you feel honestly about the situation?** Not good, no, definitely not. It was really me, being reactive and responding to my stuff, rather than looking at what was going on for that person. I was appalled actually. I have always prided myself on doing good work, and certainly that had been my history. And here I was, not able to deal with my own reactivity.

Interpreting

Interpreting involves clarifying and explaining the meaning of a communicative action situation.

- **What were my hopes for the practice outcomes in this story?** The purpose of our meetings was to support that worker in doing a really good job, in their work, and feeling like they were supported in a bureaucratic environment that wasn't easy. It was also that I would be able to work out what was going on for me, so that I could do something about it.

- **How were my hopes related to my ideals of what constitutes 'good' practice?** It wasn't good practice at all, what I did. My ideals would have been to have put my own stuff to the side, listen to it, because I think it is important to listen to your own stuff, but rather than making a comment that I think was quite judgemental of that person, I should have explored more what was going on for them, that made them see that situation in that way, what their reflection on that might be, what they felt they might need from me in exploring all of that. If I was not able to do that, I hoped that by doing my own reflective practice with someone, I would find a resolution to this situation. So, a really different response would have been my ideal.

- **What are the sources in my life and work for my ideas and values for communicative aspects of my practice?** Well, certainly my training, which includes narrative therapy, feminism, and I come from a poststructural perspective, and social justice as well. I engage in supervision, or reflective practice for myself on a regular basis with people, and I also do a lot of reflection by myself when I feel uncomfortable about how I have handled something.

- **In what ways do I embody them now in the way I communicate at work?** My feminist values help me to embody openness, fairness, being heard, listening and being there for the other. My poststructural and social justice values ensure that I am mindful of injustice and the operations of power and I want to bring that to the forefront of discussions. I want to create openings for people to explore their experiences from different perspectives. I want our conversations to find ways of acknowledging what people give value to and to review those experiences through that lens. The values I embody from narrative therapy are to do with working with people to encourage them tell their own life stories, so they can get to a place where they review those life stories.

- **What was my communicative role in this situation?** My role was to provide 'super-vision' – to help this person reflect on their situation, what it was like for them, the sense they made of it, and then work with them to help them to feel supported in doing a good job in their work.

- **To what extent did I achieve my communicative role?** In this case, I didn't do well at all. I let their comments get to me and because those comments managed to press my buttons, I acted outside of my usual values and my role of what I would usually do as a supervisor. So, I did not act according to my values terribly well, nor did I achieve my role at all well, in this case. However, those values did alert me to the fact that things had not gone so well, and prompted me to seek supervision in relation to that.

- **How did my interpretation of my role affect my relations with the people in the situation?** In this situation, even though I had hoped otherwise, I was affected by the person's comments. In my role as a supervisor I am usually very responsive to the person's needs and it all goes well. In this case, my role was affected by the comments made by the worker. I found myself becoming reactive.

- **What are the shared communication norms and expectations in this situation? In other words, how did everyone else in the story interpret their roles and what did they seem to expect in the situation?** Of myself, I think I expected to play a particular role which is to help them explore what is going on for them and to be able to access the skills and knowledge they have available to them, to add to that, if that's appropriate, to make them feel safe in the circumstance, so they can actually talk through what is going on for them. The person in this situation can usually expect to feel safe to talk, to understand what is going on and to hopefully make their situation better. This person made comments unrelated to the work situation that finally got to me and made me feel reactive. I'm not sure what that person expected of me when they made those comments. Perhaps that was part of the problem.

- **To what extent were social norms, or sets of expectations for behaviour, operating in this situation?** Normally, supervision goes well, because it is a conversation about work matters in a trusting, safe environment. In this case, the comments seemed to come from another agenda, outside of the work issue we were there to discuss.

- **What system of spoken and unspoken rewards and penalties was in place to maintain and control socially accepted behaviours in this situation?** Supervision is a professional requirement, but it is intended to be of help to the worker, to make them feel heard and helped in their work issues. Ordinarily, supervisory sessions flow easily, even though there is a professional obligation to some extent, because the process is helpful and issues are identified and addressed. As the supervisor, my role is to help and encourage through facilitating communication and reflection, but there is an obligation for the worker to attend sessions, nonetheless, and for me to act in the role of supervisor, of course. Both parties usually know and respect the way the supervision process works and they communicate accordingly. One of the things I realized after I did some reflective practice over this matter, was that there were structural and circumstantial factors which were muddying up the clarity of the role I had in this situation. This realization was very useful for me as it gave me a way of understanding better some of my own reactions.

- **Were the usual communicative norms and sanctions altered in this situation?** Yes, because the usual ebb and flow of conversation was not as easy as it is usually. I usually stay grounded and centred to facilitate sessions, but the comments this person made unsteadied me and made me reactive. I try to minimize any power potentials in conversations, but that may not always be interpreted as such by the worker. The communication norms were way off their usual trajectory.

Learning

Learning involves creating new insights and integrating them into your existing awareness and knowledge.

- **What does this scenario tell me about my expectations of myself?**

That I am human. What it basically tells me is that I don't think I can do the ideal – play the ideal role – and remain in that ideal space, with everyone under every circumstance. There are some particular situations or interactions, especially if they have built up over time, where that escapes me. Where everything that I know slips though my fingers, because I am human.

- **What does this scenario tell me about my expectations of other people?** Through that process of reflection I engaged in about this scenario, I acknowledged that at some time previously, as a professional, I had hoped to play an ideal role to some extent – that if I provided an ideal space and the communication went well, that I might reasonably expect to be of help to most people.

- **What have I learned from this situation?** Well, I don't think this is about blaming the other person in any way, shape or form, and I don't. It is much more that there are some people who I am not going to be able to meet despite my best efforts. It is not because I am good and they are bad, it is just because of the differences between us and the vulnerabilities each of us brings to these situations. Furthermore, the structural and circumstantial issues were quite significant, and were affecting both myself and this worker. I think it is really important to acknowledge that, that I can't be everything to everyone – that there are gaps in my knowledge and my life experience, things that I can never fill, just because that's the way life is.

- **What kinds of adaptations are possible in my work relationships?** It means that I don't *get* some people and that's OK, it's about recognizing that and hopefully recognizing it early enough that I don't make comments to people that leave them feeling they are put down in any way, which is really inappropriate, because it is not about that. You know, maybe someone else who comes from different life experiences, who sees the world slightly differently to me, would have been able to engage with that person really, really well. It is also about identifying those structural and circumstantial factors, and recognizing and doing something about how they are impacting on me.

- **How do I fit these new insights into my present ways of regarding communicative action in my work?** I think I adjusted my expectations, so when I explored all of that and came to that conclusion with that one, it was like: 'Oh, well maybe I need to put my expectations of what I can be and what I can do with this particular person to the side and look at where the limitations are and look at what is possible and renegotiate this relationship, so that I don't get into that place again with this person.' It is really about: 'Let's recognize where the limitations and contextual factors are to this relationship and just be up front about it,' in some way that doesn't put the other person down.

Author's reflection

When I was in my mid-twenties, I had two confronting personal experiences, which, though they were painful at the time, assisted me to alter for ever after certain entrenched communication patterns I had formed as ways of interacting with people.

The first interaction happened was when I was a member of an amateur theatre group, taking small parts in musicals. For example, I played Nettie in *Carousel* and sang 'When You Walk Through a Storm'. Our rehearsals were intense and our troupe worked hard to ensure the local people felt they had value for money in coming to one of our shows. One afternoon, I remember talking with another member of the group, a man named John. I was chattering on excitedly about something or another, I can't remember the topic. It was my tendency to fill silence with chatter, as though it was my duty to supply entertainment for any gaps in conversations. John drew breath, hesitated briefly, and then looked at me compassionately, and simply said: 'Bev, when there's nothing to say, say nothing!'

I remember a sharp stabbing sensation in my chest as his words hit home and resonated as truth. My feelings of embarrassment glowed in the redness of my face, as I became acutely aware of my tendency towards incessant babbling. In that instant, I realised his good intentions, and managed to say nothing. A bit later I had the space to think about what he said and I appreciated John's courage in delivering those wise words. I realized that my tendency for empty talkativeness came from competing for attention in my family and from sometimes having to overstate the obvious as a means of explaining my position, for fear of being misunderstood. As my life became more public and I developed skills as a practitioner and as an academic, I was grateful to John for pointing out my habitual chattering. Silence is sometimes the wisest option in complex personal and professional interactions.

The second confronting experience was delivered with a lot less grace, but it resulted in making me become conscious of and change another communication habit. I was working as a registered nurse in a Red Cross blood bank connected to a rural hospital, where local people came to donate blood. Although it was not a technically difficult procedure, I needed to undertake the venesection with care, to site the needle and monitor the blood flow, and prevent complications after donation, such as bruising or haematoma formation and fainting. I attended to many donors in a day, often working rapidly to prevent delays for people needing to get back to work after their blood donation.

On one particular day, Colleen, a registered nurse I knew as a very effective 'hot shot' practitioner, came to donate blood, and as was my habit, after the initial greeting and commencement of the procedure, I related to her in what I thought was a friendly manner. When the blood was running well into the sterile pack, I could see that she was red-faced and seemed irritable. Within a minute or so, Colleen exclaimed angrily: 'Bev, I hate the way you call everyone "love" or "darling". It is so patronizing!' I was flabbergasted at her reaction, and felt so shocked that my well-meant friendliness had made her so angry. I apologized immediately, completed the procedure carefully, and within minutes Colleen went away with less fury, but she was still angry nonetheless. We never revisited the incident and I was left to make sense of it.

On reflection, I realized that my tendency to call people 'love' and 'darling' was learned in my family, in my working-class roots, where ways of talking to one another were easy and familiar. In my workplace, I had used the same easy greetings to intend friendliness, but in a work context of many patients' admissions and discharges, they were in fact a lazy means of not having to use or remember people's actual names. I could also see that my relatively powerful position of being the person with the venesection needle in my hands was not in a working-class context of confirming my egalitarian place in my family, and that it did, in fact, reek of patronization. I was grateful to Colleen for pointing out my shortcomings in communication, even though her delivery of the message could have been more considerate.

I still call my sister, son, partner and other family and friends 'darling' and they know it is said with a heart of love. However, I now discriminate those situations where the greeting is inappropriate, so 'Thank you Colleen' for teaching me how to recognize the difference.

As a corollary, I've since realized that it is important to give and receive confronting feedback at times, but while always trying to receive feedback as gracefully as I can, I have definitely tried to emulate John's example, of delivering confronting feedback considerately.

Summary

This chapter reviewed some information connected directly to practical reflection, before guiding you through the practical reflection process. Communication is complex because it involves human beings with mixed motives and agendas. In the complexity of healthcare practice, communication becomes even more challenging. Practical reflection can assist you to make your way through the maze of human communication work. I hope you find it useful for your practice.

Key points

- Practical reflection is derived from the work of Smyth (1986a, 1986b) and Street (1991), with an adaptation to emphasize the communicative nature of this type of reflection.
- Practical reflection retains some of the questions used previously by Smyth and Street, within the process of experiencing, interpreting and learning.
- Experiencing involves retelling a practice story so that you experience it again in as much detail as possible.
- Interpreting involves clarifying and explaining the meaning of a communicative action situation.
- Learning involves creating new insights and integrating them into your existing awareness and knowledge.
- Although change may not be an explicit aim of practical reflection, it is still possible through new insights that follow from raised awareness.
- Through the medium of language, practical reflection will help you to understand the interpersonal basis of human experiences and will also offer you the potential for creating new knowledge, which interprets the meaning of your lived experience, context and subjectivity.

6 Emancipatory reflection

Introduction

This chapter reviews some information connected directly to emancipatory reflection, before guiding you through the emancipatory reflection process.

Beyond objective reasoning provided by technical reflection, and awareness and description offered by practical reflection, is a critical view of your practice and the constraints within it. If you are thwarted by the power relationships within your practice and work setting, you may need to adopt emancipatory reflective processes to bring about transformative action.

Although I am aware of the potential of emancipatory reflection to bring about positive changes, I am also very aware of the enormity of the task which faces any reflective healthcare professional who 'takes on the system' to change the status quo. In fact, I am so aware of the inherent dangers in the process that I have warned teachers of reflective practice that they should be careful about sending clinicians out prematurely to bring about change through reflective practice, without ongoing support to fight 'big battles for small gains' (Taylor 1997). With this in mind, I suggest that you find a colleague with whom to work collaboratively on your emancipatory issues. A critical friend may also be helpful, as he or she can act as a colleague, keeping you company on this journey of reflective practice.

Emancipatory reflection is only as liberating as the amount of effort you are willing to invest in making a thorough and systematic critique of the constraints within your practice. Emancipatory reflection will help you to analyse critically the contextual features which have a bearing on your practice, whether they are personal, political, sociocultural, historical or economic.

Personal constraints involve some unique features about you as a healthcare professional, into which you may or may not have insights. Political constraints are about work relationships and power struggles that happen day to day. The features of the workplace and how people define their entire ways of being together in that setting constitute sociocultural constraints. Historical constraints are those factors that have been inherited in a setting, which have the potential to cause difficulties. Economic constraints have to do with a lack of money in settings in which the health dollar is being made to stretch further and further. Healthcare practice can include some or all of these constraints, depending on particular work settings and the people interacting in them.

Emancipatory reflection is based on the work of Smyth (1986a) and Street (1991), even though they did not name the process 'emancipatory reflection' as such. Of all the types of reflection, it is the richest, but riskiest, in terms of what it tries to achieve and the courage it requires to use it effectively. It requires clinicians to make a deep, systematic and direct analysis of their work to locate the reasons effective practice is constrained. Given the hegemonic and reified conditions in work settings and relationships, this is no small task. Even so, the process has effects and rewards that can be so impressive as to change the habitual ways you define yourself and go about your daily work.

Review of previous ideas

In Chapter 3 I explained that critical knowledge is derived from some key ideas in critical social science which have the potential to be emancipatory – that is, to have freeing possibilities. In particular, critical social science has the potential to free people from the oppression of their social and personal conditions by questioning the status quo of various potentially repressive social contexts, to discover and expose the forces that maintain them for the advantages of particular people or regimes. This means that it looks at the nature of powerful relationships in life and asks how they might be different and better for the majority of people, not just for the privileged few. There are many key ideas in critical social science, but the ones included in emancipatory reflection are false consciousness, hegemony, reification, emancipation and empowerment. Many of these ideas are related, and they describe the depth and scope of forces which can keep people controlled and subordinated.

False consciousness is the 'systematic ignorance that the members of . . . society have about themselves and their society' (Fay 1987: 27). Ignorance of oppressive forces means that they remain unchallenged. Hegemony means the ascendancy or domination of one power over another, and it refers to the ways in which some social systems, and the people in them, give the impression that they are unassailable, and that the conditions they have produced are not only good, but also appropriate for the people over whom they have control. Healthcare settings have hegemonic influences operating within them that maintain false consciousness, but emancipatory reflection helps you to see where they are and how they create and maintain their power to work against you.

Fay (1987: 92) explains that reification means 'making into a thing' and he defines it as 'taking what are essential activities and treating them as if they operated according to a given set of laws independently of the wishes of the social actors who engage in them'. These laws of social life are assigned a power of their own, thus becoming accepted and unquestioned as givens. When practices become reified, they are immensely resistant to change because they are so deeply entrenched and accepted that they are embedded in the matrix of practice and thereby become relatively impervious to identification and critique.

Emancipation means freedom, from your own and from other people's expectations and roles, and to adopt other self-aware and socially aware practices. Empowerment is the process of giving and accepting power, to liberate people from their oppressive circumstances. Emancipatory reflection alerts you to the possibilities of emancipation and gives you the means to empower yourself and others.

In summary, critical knowledge is potentially liberating for individuals and groups of people, when they realize that they may be living under misunderstandings about themselves and their social situations – misunderstandings which have been developed and held systematically. As people and practitioners, healthcare professionals are subject to oppressive social structures which can be transformed through critical analysis and action. Emancipatory interest is rooted in power and creates 'transformative action' which seeks to provide emancipation from forces which limit people's rational control of their lives. These forces are so influential and taken for granted that people have the strong impression that they are beyond their control.

Emancipatory reflection involves human interaction, but it emphasizes how people interpret themselves within their roles and social obligations. Emancipatory reflection leads to 'transformative action', which seeks to free you from your taken-for-granted assumptions and oppressive forces which limit you and your practice. Emancipatory reflection provides you with a systematic means of critiquing the status quo in the power relationships in your workplace and offers you raised awareness and a new sense of informed consciousness to bring about positive social and political change. It also offers you freedom from your own misguided and firmly held perceptions of yourself and your roles, to bring about change for the better. The process for change is *praxis*, which offers clinicians the means for change through collaborative processes that analyse and challenge existing forces and distortions brought about by the dominating effects of power in human interaction.

Reflector

How do you define a 'good day' at work? Do you identify a day at work as 'good' because it is unremarkable in the sense that not much goes wrong? If this is so, look closely at your 'good day' and see whether it contains unexamined issues of power. If you are alerted to the practices involved in a 'good day', you may uncover aspects of your work that have become hidden and silenced through hegemonic influences.

Practice story

Ruth is an occupational therapist in her late fifties, who related a practice story in Chapter 5 involving difficulties in communication at work. In this practice story Ruth reflects on a work issue involving unequal power relations, which are rich sources for emancipatory reflection.

This client had a long-term chronic illness; multiple sclerosis (MS). He was a single male of non-Australian origin, of different religion and ethnic background to most Australians, although it is common now. He was a very well educated, eloquent man with very good English, who chose Australia and an alternate lifestyle, and this was the difficulty. He liked to design things himself and prescribe for himself how he was to manage. Part of it might have been the euphoria accompanying MS at times, but he did have his own, explicit ideas. Over the years, it was difficult. With MS, the spasm and lack of control of the limbs makes certain things dangerous, such as cooking, handling boiling water, which he insisted on doing against my and caregivers' recommendations. He would make coffee for himself and frequently burned himself, so that didn't go well.

He had very poor hygiene when I became involved. He needed showering a lot more and he totally refused. So, he was exercising his power over the carers. And there were transfer issues, which became very complicated. He made up his own transfer device, which was a log of wood swinging from the ceiling. So, he very much wanted to be self empowered in what he needed. The clashes came then with caregivers; the right of a person to choose versus the duty of care. Frequently, the caregivers would ring me and say: 'This is not working'. He would not allow a case manager, but when it came to functional issues within the home, such as safety, then it came back to me to manage. The manager of the caregivers at the time was intolerant of this client's behaviour and choices, would rather not have him as a client, but had to, by law, but looked down on him. He did not accept this client's rights as an individual, so I came up against that.

The caregivers were always safe, however, I was brought in several times with: 'Please assess this transfer business', that is, he was not using the equipment provided, rather he was using the log of wood hanging from the ceiling. It was bolted into the rafters. I certainly did not approve it. His hygiene was so poor that the carers' hygiene was being threatened, such as with faeces, not to mention that the entire unit had urine in the carpet and the smell was rank. The bedding was rank as well and sometimes he refused for the bedding to be changed. He came in from out in the bush from a shared living commune into a Department of Housing unit in town. He didn't work much, only enough to pay for food and his food was very basic, but quite nutritious – he was never emaciated. He wanted that hippie lifestyle in the Department of Housing unit, hence the log hanging from the ceiling and so on. His lifestyle was a little bit more primitive and it might have been all right on floorboards in his previous home, but the urine soaked into the carpet in his unit in town.

The next issue was his insistence on living alone – if he had been admitted to a nursing home he would have been assessed for a high level of care – however, he was still living in the community, alone. He was trying to feed himself with 'Meals on Wheels' and drink hot fluids. He gave up wearing clothes, because he couldn't get undressed and he was wearing a T-shirt, which was often dirty. We had changing caregivers who liked to do their best, but it was really difficult for them to provide adequate service because the client refused, because of his need for self-empowerment. Then, I would come in and make a recommendation. In the first few years the client nearly always rejected it.

He was unrealistic of his abilities – he drove a car, which was a nightmare. Eventually he stopped driving – it took a long time. We did not report him to the police. He had control of the steering wheel, but his lower limbs went into spasm and it was a manual car. He drove himself about 1,400 kilometres to another city and he had such pressure wounds on his heels that he had them dressed. He had neuropathy and he couldn't feel it, so his heels were really badly affected. The professionals who dressed the wounds said: 'We really think you need hospitalization with those heels.' He said: 'Well, I'm not going to hospital here.' So, he got in the car and returned to this area, which is a three-day drive. We think he called into an emergency department on the way and had the dressing changed and when he arrived back here, he was admitted, with these terrible wounds. This is how unrealistic he was and so self-empowered, that hospitals could not intervene.

After the wounds healed he went back home, and he refused home care at the time, but he accepted it some time later. He was admitted to hospital some time later and then we had the dictatorial approach of the hospital – not so much the nurses – but I heard him being abused by a wardsman. I just happened to hear it from the next room. I thought: 'No, let's try to get him out'. I just made up my mind to try to get him out of hospital to protect him. This client would never complain, ever, and the wardsman could not understand that he had extensor spasm and could not bend his knees, and I thought: 'This could happen in a nursing home as well'. So, I wanted to get him home.

I got all the stakeholders together for a case conference. I put it to him: 'Do you want to go home?' He said: 'Yes'. I said: 'You must accept my recommendations for your care, so that this situation does not occur again. If you get care at home when you need it, will you accept these conditions?' And he said: 'Yes'. That was the first time he ever submitted to a condition, ever. I was rather passionate to get him home and it took only seven days. 'If you want this, you will need seven days of personal care, because you smell,' I finally told him, because I had been reluctant to insult him, but I was able to do this and he accepted everything I said. I got the continence adviser in and the community nurse and the home care.

We came to a verbal agreement with the client about the care interventions. I had a camera and when we took him home we videoed how the care would be done, for example, the transfers with a hoist, so the log would no longer be used. The incontinence was managed. I filmed everything except that (the incontinence management) – how to do the transfers, how to use the wheelchair and store it, the placement of the telephone, chairs, bed. The incontinence management was his private business with the nurses. We were able to move his heavy timber frame king-size bed. We filmed all the procedures and it was made available for caregivers to see what we had agreed on, because of changing caregivers to ensure continuity of care. Not only that, I filmed his agreement because he could not write. 'Do you agree to the filming?' 'Yes.' 'Do you agree it takes two people to handle you?' 'Yes, I agree.' So, I was able to film that agreement. He was totally cooperative and very happy with the outcome.

It took years to establish that rapport, and for him to trust me and agree with my recommendations. It took years for the rapport and him valuing what I can offer. He had to see that I was doing it for him, that it was not for me, at all, it was for him. Because that was something I valued, that he had right of choice. My value was to get him home, where I knew he wanted to be, even though I knew he really needed 24/7 nursing home type care. I valued his rights for independence with as much choice as I could offer him, whereas there were other powers that would have liked to disempower him. I guess I became passionate to support him.

The value about being passionate to support came from my mother, who was a strong force for independence. She was my role model. The clients I see cannot always have a high level of independence, but wherever possible I will try to provide it. My background was about independence and self-empowerment – the right to choose your lifestyle. But I have to introduce modifications to lifestyles, which a lot of people don't like. They sometimes reject it, but gradually accept it after years of:

'Well, if you do it like this, this will happen'. My work is client focused, always. 'Where are you? What are you doing? Why do you need to do this and this? Show me.'

When I do a home visit, it's their home, not mine. I am a guest. I am fortunate to be able to be accepted at the front door and that's the way I respect it. I respect clients and their domain. Even though I have expertise in, say, transfer techniques and home modifications, this is their home. They may reject my ideas and say: 'No, I want it this way'. I've learnt to be more patient with people making decisions, to enable them to make their own. In this case, with the client whose story I have been relating, there was no live-in caregiver and I didn't have to deal with anyone else. I've learned to be more patient and try to respect them and to put things, such as strategies, in ways that they can understand. In this case, the client was unreasonable, so I had to reword things.

I've also learned from this practice experience the progress of some degenerative diseases. Because I have been working so long, I can see from the start to the end stage. I've seen people who've gone home, who shouldn't have gone home, because of the pressure on the families. I've seen things go wrong. I've been able to learn the long-term needs of people and I know what to expect and sometimes I've been asked to advise in that way: 'What can we expect?' Sometimes I have tentatively told people what they might need, what might happen. I don't like doing that too often though, because I am not God, I can't predict. It makes me aware with some patients with degenerative diseases that they are not going to get better. I also have to think of the house they are living in – of what I've seen with this client. Will I let it go this far? Will I intervene beforehand? How soon will I intervene with the heavy equipment or major modifications?

Summary

This section revisited some key ideas relating to emancipatory reflection and shared Ruth's practice story, to show the complexity of her occupational therapy practice, especially when power plays are operating. The next section introduces you to the process of emancipatory reflection, before demonstrating the approach with a worked clinical example.

The process of emancipatory reflection

Daily work incidents are imbued with power. If you look closely, you will begin to see subtle and not so subtle examples of power plays within healthcare settings that are taken for granted as 'just the way things are'. Emancipatory reflection provides a process to construct, confront, deconstruct and reconstruct your practice. *Construction* of practice incidents allows you to describe, in words and other creative images and representations, a work scene played out previously, bringing to mind all the aspects and constraints of the situation. *Deconstruction* involves asking analytical questions regarding the situation, which are aimed at locating and critiquing all the aspects. *Confrontation* occurs when you focus on your part in the scenario with the intention of seeing and describing it as clearly as possible. *Reconstruction* puts the scenario together again with transformative strategies for managing changes in the light of the new insights.

There are many constraints operating in work settings, including cultural, economic, historical, political, social and personal (see Chapter 1), which may affect the ways in which you are able to interpret and act at any given moment.

Reflector

What are the practice constraints in your profession? How do they stop you from practising effectively? What kinds of constraint operate at subtle levels in your workplace? How can you recognize them? What effects do they have on your practice?

You are a central character in your practice stories, reflecting on your own practice as it relates to other people and determinants of the situation. When you have reflected on one scenario, you can go on to reflect on as many as you choose. Keep a record of all your reflections; they will be interesting to compare, because they track your reflective journey, and they will show you your main issues and how you are working through them using reflective processes.

Choose an incident in which you were not entirely happy about the outcomes of your involvement, that is, you felt that you did not make a difference of a positive nature to someone in your care. The incident should also exemplify an imbalance of power and cooperation between people. The situation can involve as many people as you like, but you should be central in the activity. The following steps guide you through the reflective writing processes of construction, to describe the situation as fully as possible.

Constructing

In order to construct an incident in which you felt that you did not make a difference of a positive nature and there was an imbalance of power and cooperation, it might help to shut your eyes and take yourself back in your imagination to that time. You could also use other strategies to enhance your memory, such as those described in Chapter 2. When you have a clear image of the situation, write down, or represent creatively, a full description of the experience. If you respond to the following questions you will be able to build up a 'thick description' of the event:

- What was happening?
- When was it happening?
- Where was it happening?
- What was the setting like, in terms of its smells, sounds and sights?
- Why was it happening?
- Who was involved?
- How were you involved?
- What were the outcomes of the situation?
- How did you feel honestly about the situation?

Now you need to review your construction of the situation:

- Is your description or creative representation as rich and full as possible?
- Does it capture the scene as faithfully as possible?

You might like to go back and elaborate further to ensure that you have described the experience as well as you possibly can. As you may have noticed already, a rich and full description at the outset provides more information on which to reflect.

Deconstructing

If you have been able to capture the context, you should have before you a fully descriptive scenario of the interactions and inherent power relations in an aspect of your practice. The reason I have described power relations as 'inherent' is that they will be there, but they may not be explicit at this point, especially as this story may not be able to capture all of the people's intentions and behaviours. Even if you use this process to describe a story in which events appear to go well, there may be implicit power plays operating. A critical view of practice helps you to see the power relations which bubble away, possibly just under the surface of what is apparent immediately. With this in mind, revisit your account or creative representation and see what you can locate in terms of political motives and outcomes.

Identify your involvement in the scenario by looking at your part with the eyes of an interested observer standing back from the action. When you locate aspects of your contributions to the interaction, investigate your motives and actions by musing tentatively: 'It seems as if I act according to my belief that . . .' By completing this sentence as often as you need to, you will find the stimuli in practice that 'push your buttons' and make you react each time they come up in some form or another. The chances are that you will find these themes in your reflection, even though initially your practice stories appear to have little relation to one another.

Express yourself as clearly as you can, so that your observing self-identifies, frankly and honestly, the person you have represented as yourself in the scenario. Write down or audiotape any observations you make, so that you can revisit them. Alternatively, you might like to write poetry or use some other creative means to respond to this part of the process. At this point, however, you need to be as clear in your mind as possible about what your musing means, so you need to make a note of your responses and interpret your creative reflections as they 'speak' to you.

Confronting

To become aware critically you need to remain vigilant and take a critical view of practice. Even when situations appear relatively positive, power interests may mediate them. To confront these power issues you need to ask questions such as:

- Where did the ideas I embody in my practice come from historically?
- How did I come to appropriate them? In other words, how did I take them on?
- Why do I continue now to endorse them in my work?
- Whose interests do they serve?
- What power relations are involved?
- How do these ideas influence my relationships with the people in my care?
- What cultural, economic, historical, political, social and/or personal constraints are operating in this practice story (adapted from Smyth 1986a)?

In being prepared to ask these questions, you are making a critical analysis of your practice world. You will begin to see that even though you are often at the centre of your world, you are certainly not the only determinant of the situation. The world in which you exist and act is influenced by historical, sociocultural, economic and political determinants, which to greater and lesser extents constrain the ways in which you are free to interpret and act in any given moment. The realization that you are 'not alone' in your practice can free you from bitter self-recriminations and raise the possibilities of new awareness. At some stage it may also be possible to transform the repressive conditions which cause you to act in certain ways.

Reconstructing

Reconstructing puts the scenario together again with transformative strategies for managing changes in the light of new insights. Given that you have been able to follow the process of systematic inquiry outlined so far, by now you may have realized that there may be contradictions in what you *say* you think, say and do, and what you *actually* think, say and do.

The only remaining step in the process is to free yourself to the possibilities of using your raised awareness in reconstructing your world. There may be a lot of time, space and effort between raised awareness and change, but if you do not allow yourself to imagine the possibilities of transformation, then nothing will be possible. If you dare to imagine and to plan to act in ways that are capable of transforming your world, then you will have attempted to break free from the taken-for-granted assumptions which maintain the status quo.

The final question to be posed is:

- In the light of what I have discovered, how might I work differently?

As you imagine some different ways of acting, don't forget that you are not alone in your work setting. Consider how historical, sociocultural, economic and political determinants might play a part in the way you are able to work. Begin to imagine or make some adjustments to some of the situational constraints as part of your plan of action for change.

An example of emancipatory reflection

Jenny, aged 38, is an experienced nurse with 15 years experience in acute nursing care, and in the last five years she been in a senior nursing management position that has allowed her to keep her clinical proficiency while influencing practice management. As such, Jenny is a respected member of the healthcare team, especially the nurses, who often ask her to assist them in solving complex clinical problems. Her clinical nursing and management role also requires her to communicate often with doctors in forming clinical guidelines for procedures.

Jenny is also a member of a reflective practice group, which is using action research to work through the clinical issue of the need for assertion, especially in situations in which there are power imbalances. Jenny told her practice story about meeting with two doctors to look at possible changes to some clinical guidelines.

Constructing

- **What? When? Where? Why? What was the setting like? Who was involved? How were you involved?** As part of my role as the clinical nurse manager, I had to meet with two doctors during the week. The intention of the meeting was to review the present guidelines for emergency resuscitation and to make any changes that might be necessary in the light of new research-based evidence for best practice. We met in one of the rooms in the education centre around 1 p.m., and the meeting was to last for around an hour or so. It was quiet and private in the room and with only three of us in the subcommittee I felt outnumbered as the only nurse.

- **What were the outcomes of the situation?** All seemed to be going well until the doctors bamboozled me with generic names of recently marketed drugs. I know the names of most drugs, of course, but I don't always use their generic names for simplicity's sake. Some new drugs have come onto the market recently, but they are not necessarily in common use in hospital settings as yet. They began talking among themselves as though I was not there. Their tactic effectively silenced me and I was unable to contribute much after that, because they kept the subject on medications, rather than sticking to the task of reviewing the entire procedure, not just the drug therapies.

- **How did you feel honestly about the situation?** I honestly felt as though it was a case of 'We'll show this hot-shot nurse! Thinks she's smart, does she?' I felt like it was two against one and I felt overwhelmed and outnumbered. I also felt patronized and I felt that they were trying to get rid of me, as inconsequential to any decisions they might make.

Deconstructing

A member of the reflective practice group asked Jenny to identify her involvement in the scenario by looking at her part with the eyes of an interested observer standing back from the action. Jenny located aspects of her contributions to the interaction by investigating her motives and actions and musing tentatively: 'It seems as if I act according to my belief that . . .' By completing this sentence often she found some of the stimuli in her practice that 'push her buttons' and make her react each time they come up in some form or another.

Jenny said: 'It seems as if I act according to my belief that doctors should respect nurses' knowledge and skills. I was indignant that these doctors used the generic names to keep me out of the conversation and to silence me. Therefore, following on from that, it seems as if I value being part of a multidisciplinary team, but I don't really feel like an equal in it. Also, by remaining silent because of their exclusion tactics, it seems as if I am willing to comply with their dominance over me. Possibly, somewhere deep inside me I must hold the thought that doctors know more than me and that they have the power when it comes to multidisciplinary teams, despite all the rhetoric we perpetuate that we all contribute as equals in multidisciplinary teams, such as in this committee.'

Confronting

Jenny knew that to become aware critically she needed to remain vigilant and take a critical view of her practice. To confront the power issues she responded to the following questions:

- **Where did the ideas I embody in my practice come from historically?** From my practice story I can see that I value the ideas of respect, collaboration and equality. Historically these values come from growing up in a large family, having to share and cooperate with one another. As I became an adult I realized that valuing respect, collaboration and equality were good markers for life, so I have continued to uphold them. Even so, this story shows me that I also embody passivity to power, that is, in the face of lack of respect, collaboration and equality, I do not necessarily always assert my right for these values to be honoured or reciprocated.
- **How did I come to appropriate them?** I took on the ideas of respect, collaboration and equality as I developed expertise and confidence in my work relations. Most of the time I actively embody them in my relationships with people at work, but sometimes they are not that obvious in my practice.
- **Why do I continue now to endorse them in my work?** I continue to endorse respect, collaboration and equality now in my practice, because they work for me most of the time, and they help me to work as an effective multidisciplinary team member. I suppose I feel that if I embody these values I might become a role model for other people. This means that if I show other people how to be respectful, and to work collaboratively and with equality, they might catch on and treat me and other people in the same way. Widely spread across the entire organization, respect, collaboration and equality can only have good effects that are advantageous for everyone.
- **Whose interests do they serve?** They are positive values that should ideally serve everyone's interests, in that they form a good foundation for relating to one another in the multidisciplinary team. I must admit also, that they serve my purposes because if I can model them, they might flow back to me and make my work life a lot happier. Just imagine, if people in

power in the hierarchy embodied these values, there would be less 'grandstanding', egos would be in check, and it would take a lot of anxiety away from me, if I could come to work each day and know everyone was enacting their roles with respect, collaboration and equality.

- **What power relations are involved?** Respect, collaboration and equality do not work when everyone in the multidisciplinary team does not value or embody them, and this is demonstrated very well in my story, when doctors used language to hammer home their clinical superiority. They used their medical power over me to obliterate any possibility of respect, collaboration and equality. In fact, I could go so far as to say that they sensed my willingness to embody these values and took advantage of me, because of them. In other words, sensing my willingness to be respectful and to collaborate on equal terms with them, they seized that as their opportunity to turn the situation around to their advantage, and to make me look weak and passive for trying to embody these values.

- **How do these ideas influence my relationships with the people in my care?** They influence my work relationships by giving me some values on which to make my decisions and act ethically, in relation to the people with whom I come into contact. For example, I care for my patients with these values in mind – they deserve my respect and we collaborate in the planning of their care, as equals in terms of our shared humanity. Patients may look to me to have extra knowledge and skills that they do not possess, but that does not mean that I use that expertise to talk down to them, or treat them like lesser beings.

- **What cultural, economic, historical, political, social and/or personal constraints are operating in this practice story?** Let's see – in my practice story about the doctors using their knowledge as power over me, I consider that the cultural constraints operating between us had to do with how we see ourselves in terms of the symbols and rituals that denote our different practices. For example, doctors use medical language as a device to maintain distance and to exert authority and superiority. While I may have considerable skills in speaking in medical terminology, and I am able to decode the vast majority of it, in my story these doctors used their knowledge of recently marketed generic drug names to intentionally leave me behind in the conversation. That left me with the alternatives to speak up and ask for a decoding or translation of their medical language, or to remain silent. I was feeling patronized and I did not want to give them the satisfaction of knowing that their cultural strategy to distance and exclude me from the conversation had in fact worked. There were no economic constraints operating in this situation that I can see. Economic constraints happen often in clinical settings, but not in this case. Rare, isn't it! The historical constraints are those that we have perpetuated from long ago, when doctors were indisputable 'lords of the manor' and no one dared to question that. Historically, doctors have enjoyed a great deal of professional power in the hospital hierarchy and some still hanker for those days when their word was not questioned and we nurses ran around willingly as handmaidens to them. Times have changed and we now acknowledge other professionals' knowledge and expertise by forming multidisciplinary teams. However, history holds a strong influence over the present day and some doctors may not have moved on much from being the dominant member of the health team. Nurses have historically come from a tradition of subservience to doctors and I realize that my response to these doctors shows me that the constraints of history still have an influence on me. The political constraints were the power and prestige differences, acted out by two doctors shutting out one nurse, in a political manoeuvre managed through language. Professional politics are not always explicit I know, but in this case it was a blatant attempt to put me in my place. I'm sure they felt they were totally capable of revising the resuscitation guidelines without any help from a lowly nurse, even if she is the best nurse this hospital can offer! The social constraints are how we relate to one another as people and professionals, within the hierarchy. I am sure that these doctors did not see me as their social equal. They enjoy far higher salaries than me, drive around in luxury cars, live in the best suburbs, are members of the best clubs, stay within their own social circles and maintain their social distance by not associating with nurses outside working hours. These factors all act as constraints in a work setting in which there is rhetoric about the equal contributions of members of the multidisciplinary health team. Of course they do not see me as their equal – not in any way – culturally, historically, politically or socially. The personal constraints relate to my inability to rise above the patronizing exclusion tactics of these doctors, to assert myself in that situation. I am a shy person by nature, even though my clinical expertise gives me confidence at work. Sometimes the shy and passive person comes out at work, because it is easier and less confronting to remain silent when the stakes are high and political forces are blatantly active in clinical situations.

In being prepared to ask these questions, Jenny began to see that even though she was at the centre of this story, she was not the only determinant of the outcome. She realized that the unsatisfactory outcome was more than from her personal inability to make the situation better, rather it related to the constraints operating in this situation, such as the historical, sociocultural and political factors.

Reconstructing

Jenny realized that there were contradictions in what she said she thought and embodied, and what she actually thought, said and did. She realized that she espoused the values of respect, collaboration and equality, but it was not always possible to live by these values at work, nor was there much hope of seeing them enacted and reciprocated routinely in her work setting. She was then ready to take the final step in the process of emancipatory reflection, to free herself to the possibilities of using her raised awareness in reconstructing her practice world.

The final question Jenny posed to herself was: 'In the light of what I have discovered, how might I work differently?' Jenny reflected that in future cases of this nature, when she becomes aware of power tactics to silence her, it might be possible to speak up and ask for more information, for example: 'Could you please tell me the medications to which you are referring?' This will require her to be honest and to risk feeling vulnerable, but the sincere attempt to open up dialogue and clarify meaning could also be interpreted as mature communication embodying her values of respect, collaboration and equality among professionals.

Jenny decided that if she has a good sense of what may come up as points of discussion in similar meetings with doctors or other members of the multidisciplinary team, she could spend more time preparing herself by reviewing clinical knowledge to make her ready for most contingencies. This might mean spending time reading recent research and literature, or discussing complex ideas or new treatment regimes with peers, to make her conversant with the latest thinking in specific areas.

Jenny imagined that in situations in which the main focus of the meeting is being circumvented by other people's power agendas, she could try getting the discussion back on focus by identifying the diversion and reminding the other people of the primary intention of the conversation. This kind of assertive communication takes courage, but it is nevertheless a communication skill that can be used intentionally and with success when discussions are digressing from the main focus.

Jenny also decided that it might be appropriate sometimes to respond to a politically overwhelming situation with an assertion of her own expertise and the professional credibility she brings to the discussion. For example: 'As a nurse with X years of experience in Y, I have the responsibility for Z. Therefore, I am well placed to offer advice on A, B and C.'

Author's reflection

When I think about power plays I have experienced in practice settings, I realize that the situations that have given me the most angst over the years are not so much the ones that were 'full on, in my face' politics, because I could see them coming. No, the power plays I've put more reflection into over the years are the subtle forms of politics, such as insidious undermining, jealousy and betrayal, faint praise and so on. It's not so much that I have been dull to the various nuances in power relations in clinical settings and academia in general, rather, I just haven't seen some things coming until they were right in my face, or I have eventually felt a 'stab' in my back.

I've given it a lot of thought and I've come to a possible, tentative conclusion that my relative unpreparedness for subtler forms of work politics has been due, in part, to my tendency to keep a relatively rosy view on life and to see my glass as half full. I suspect that, had I been more willing to be more sceptical in my personality and in my dealings with people in organizations overall, I may have been more forearmed and noticed conspiracies and indirect attacks a fair bit sooner.

When I was first introduced to critical social science, which underlies emancipatory reflection, there seemed to be a huge emphasis on problematizing practices, by taking a sceptical view of people's motives and being aware of various constraining forces. This theoretical 'negativity' was noted by a colleague at the time, who made the observation that: 'Critical social science is a dismal science.' I agreed then and now, but I also am grateful that after constructing, confronting, and deconstructing comes *reconstructing*, which offers positive changes and chances of transformation. So, I guess that I'll always be a bit of a Pollyanna, and continue to get surprises when subtler forms of politics catch me unawares, but I can take heart in realizing that, should I need it, I can use a series of critical questions, like those in this emancipatory reflection approach, to help me unpack power plays, to learn from them and to bring about some changes.

Summary

This chapter reviewed some information connected directly to emancipatory reflection, before guiding you through the emancipatory reflection process. Healthcare professionals work in settings that are replete with cultural, economic, historical, political and social constraints, all of which may contrive to make your practice less than you might ideally envision. When you are thwarted by constraints and the power relationships within your practice and work setting, you can choose to adopt emancipatory reflective processes to bring about transformative action. By working through the process systematically, you may find yourself realizing that personal constraints are not the only determinants of situational outcomes and that it is possible to construct, confront, deconstruct and reconstruct your practice.

Key points

- If you are thwarted by the power relationships within your practice and work setting, you can adopt emancipatory reflective processes to bring about transformative action.
- Emancipatory reflection is only as liberating as the amount of effort you are willing to invest in making a thorough and systematic critique of the constraints within your practice.
- Emancipatory reflection will help you to analyse critically the contextual features which have a bearing on your practice, whether they are personal, political, sociocultural, historical or economic.
- Of all the types of reflection, emancipatory reflection is the richest, but riskiest, in terms of what it tries to achieve and the courage it requires to use it effectively.
- Emancipatory reflection leads to 'transformative action', which seeks to free you from your taken-for-granted assumptions and the oppressive forces which limit you and your practice.
- Emancipatory reflection provides you with a systematic means of critiquing the status quo in the power relationships in your workplace and offers you raised awareness and a new sense of informed consciousness to bring about positive social and political change.
- The process of emancipatory reflection for change is praxis, which offers clinicians the means for change through collaborative processes that analyse and challenge existing forces and distortions.
- Emancipatory reflection provides a process to construct, confront, deconstruct and reconstruct your practice.
- Construction of practice incidents allows you to describe, in words and other creative images and representations, a work scene played out previously, bringing to mind all the aspects and constraints of the situation.
- Deconstruction involves asking analytical questions regarding the situation, which are aimed at locating and critiquing all the aspects of that situation.
- Confrontation occurs when you focus on your part in the scenario with the intention of seeing and describing it as clearly as possible.
- Reconstruction puts the scenario together again with transformative strategies for managing changes in the light of the new insights.

7 Applying Taylor's REFLECT model to practice

Introduction

In Chapter 2, I introduced you to the 'Taylor model of reflection' as an easy guide to systematic reflection. The model (see Figure 2.1) is based on a mnemonic device using the word REFLECT to represent Readiness, Exercising thought, Following systematic processes, Leaving oneself open to answers, Enfolding insights, Changing awareness and Tenacity in maintaining reflection. I also demonstrated the use of the model with a practice issue experienced by Kyah, a physiotherapist, who discussed it with Kate, her critical friend.

If you have been reading this book sequentially, you have been introduced to all of the foundational ideas and technical, practical and emancipatory reflection, in Chapters 4, 5 and 6 respectively, thus you are forearmed with the information you need to become a reflective practitioner. This chapter encourages you to apply the REFLECT model to your own healthcare practice, so that you can become accustomed to reflecting on your own practice stories, in order to make sense of them and make any necessary changes. Bearing in mind the busyness of healthcare professionals, I am presenting the model in an abbreviated, point form guide (see Figure 7.1), which you can use easily and comprehensively in your workplace or at home.

Applying Taylor's REFLECT model of reflection

As a busy healthcare professional, the success you may enjoy in using any reflective process may ultimately lie in being able to bring it to mind and undertake it with ease when you are working, or when you have a chance to reflect systematically after work. When you become conversant with a particular reflective approach, it can become part of your daily repertoire as a healthcare professional. To this end, this section provides an abbreviated guide to using the REFLECT model, based on the information described in the previous chapters of this book.

When you use the guide to the Taylor model of reflection, remember that the time you take in reflecting may vary, according to your circumstances. For example, the entire REFLECT process may take only a few minutes, when you are in action at work and the issue is relatively urgent, requiring rapid reflection and action. If the REFLECT process is applied to fairly straightforward practice issues, some of the process phases may take microseconds. At other times, your practice stories may be complex with deeply entrenched issues and habits, which require hours of focused reflection at home.

With increasing levels of expertise as a professional and experience as a reflective practitioner, you may come to embody the REFLECT process to such a high degree that you become unaware of your continually engaged reflective attitude, and in unpacking a practice story later you may realize that you have actually used seemingly effortless and systematic reflective approaches in your practice most of the time.

R

Process	Activities	Reflective practitioner's notes
Readiness	Being silent Centring Setting the intention Having some reflective knowledge and skills Taking and making time Making the effort Being determined Having courage Knowing how to use humour	

E

Process	Activities	Reflective practitioner's notes
Exercising thought	Thinking on experiences Using inspiring and guiding strategies Being spontaneous Expressing freely Remaining open to ideas Choosing a time and place Being prepared personally Choosing suitable reflective methods	

F

Process	Activities	Reflective practitioner's notes
Following systematic processes	Using technical reflection: assessing planning implementing evaluating Using practical reflection: experiencing interpreting learning Using emancipatory reflection: constructing deconstructing confronting reconstructing Choosing a specific type or combination of types of reflection	

L

Process	Activities	Reflective practitioner's notes
Leaving oneself open to answers	Not jumping to early conclusions Being prepared for twists and turns Finding tentative, multiple answers Living with uncertainty	

E

Process	Activities	Reflective practitioner's notes
Enfolding insights	Mixing new insights into present understandings Using a variety of group or individual reflective processes Enlisting critical friendships Letting insights rest a while Merging into deeper and more meaningful possibilities	

C

Process	Activities	Reflective practitioner's notes
Changing awareness	Making small, manageable changes in preference to no changes at all Examining the emotional content of practice stories	

T

Process	Activities	Reflective practitioner's notes
Tenacity in maintaining reflection	Affirming yourself as a reflective practitioner Responding to the critiques Creating a daily habit Seeing things freshly Staying alert to practice Finding support systems Sharing reflection Getting involved in research Embodying reflective practice	

Figure 7.1   Guide for using Taylor's REFLECT model

Summary

This section has provided you with an abbreviated guide to using the REFLECT model, so that you can access and use it easily and comprehensively for reflecting during or after practice. I suggested that you keep in mind that the time you take in reflecting may vary from microseconds, to minutes, to hours, according to your circumstances. The ultimate hope is that with increasing levels of expertise as a professional and experience as a reflective practitioner, you come to embody the REFLECT process and become unaware of your continually engaged reflective attitude.

Writing your own practice stories

Even though you may have already been writing your own practice stories, this is an excellent opportunity to 'pull all the loose ends together' and begin to compile a portfolio of practice stories. As you are already aware, you don't necessarily have to *write* practice stories, because you can choose to record them through other creative means (see Chapter 2). A compilation of many practice stories allows you to see trends and patterns across various clinical situations, giving you clues as to the types of issues that tend to 'press your buttons'.

Reflector

Using the abbreviated REFLECT guide and other information provided in this book, reflect on at least six different clinical situations in which you have been involved directly. The situations can be from your past or present work circumstances. What trends and patterns can you discern in the stories? What practice issues surface often for you? To what extent has the REFLECT model helped you? What adaptations can you make to your reflective approaches to make reflection more useful for you and your healthcare setting?

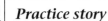

Practice story

John, aged 38, was well known as an aged care expert. He had practised and researched aged care nursing for 16 years, and was often called on by the local university to give guest lectures and act as a clinical supervisor for nursing undergraduates gaining aged care experience in the clinical area. Even so, he had only just embarked on systematic approaches to his own practice and was aware of how much he had to learn in this area. To enhance his learning, John decided to enrol in a postgraduate course in reflective practice offered by the university. As part of that learning experience, he commenced a critical friendship with a senior lecturer at the university, skilled in assisting his reflective practice experiences. John worked through a clinical issue with his critical friend, Rachael, using the systematic flow of the REFLECT model.

John reflected on a clinical situation in which he had been caring for a woman, Elsie, aged 92. Elsie had often expressed the wish to die, as she was very frail and succumbed to frequent chest infections, needing treatment at the aged care unit where John works. John became very close emotionally to Elsie over her successive admissions, and they often enjoyed conversations when Elsie was recovering. On this admission, however, Elsie was not recovering as usual after antibiotic therapy, and

John was concerned that this might be her final admission. He shared his concerns with Rachael in a one-to-one meeting at the aged care centre.

Critical friend response

John: *So, where do I start with reflection?*
Rachael: *Well, when going on a journey of discovery, you need some preparation, by getting ready.*
John: *What do I do?*
Rachael: *Nothing.*
John: *Nothing? What do you mean?*
Rachael: *Just be silent for a while. Sit in quietness for a few moments and then we'll begin.*

After a few moments of silence, John's practice story continued. He explained to Rachael that until this point in his career he had not given much thought to regular reflection. It was not as though he did not practise thoughtfully – he did – but his thinking had been mostly reactive and ad hoc, with a tendency to jump to quick and easy answers. He asked Rachael about the kind of thinking that was necessary for successful reflection.

Rachael: *When you think, what do you do?*
John: *I don't get what you mean.*
Rachael: *Imagine you are watching yourself think. What are you doing?*
John: *Nothing much. It's not as if I can see my thinking processes, but when I try to imagine it, I can see that my thoughts are often all over the place, without a lot of order and intention.*
Rachael: *Often we are unaware of thinking, so we tend to think randomly, in reaction to situations. When we exercise thought intentionally in reflection, we direct our attention to thought and make it purposeful.*

Practice story

John followed the REFLECT process to share his story about Elsie with Rachael. John responded to the questions raised in the process. He reflected as follows.

It was about 4 p.m. I had been in charge on the afternoon shift for a few hours and everything was fairly quiet. We had enough staff for our shift and the patients were settled and many of them were enjoying visits from their relatives. I could smell the aroma of the evening soup coming up from the kitchen below, there was a low hum of conversation in many of the rooms, and all seemed to be well with the world.

Elsie was in a room near the nurses' desk, because she was having IV antibiotics and we needed to keep a close eye on her, because she was especially dyspnoeic this admission. I knew Elsie very well. We became friends over the years, as she was admitted often for treatment for recurrent chest infections. I had also got to know Elsie's family, especially her grandson, Keith, who was a man in his fifties. Keith always accompanied Elsie into hospital, and he was most faithful in visiting her daily. Keith's parents lived 100 kilometres south and visited Elsie as often as they could, but Keith was Elsie's mainstay.

I went into Elsie's room and Keith was sitting lovingly beside her bed. Elsie was having intranasal low flow oxygen and the IV was running on time. Elsie raised her arm weakly and beckoned me to her side, and whispered: 'Johnny, I am out of puff. I can't go on like this. I'm an old lady Johnny. Let me die.' I was so overcome with emotion that tears flowed down my face. I have never cried in front of a patient or relative before.

Critical friend response

As John told the story his eyes glistened. He went on to say that Elsie died peacefully the next day, with Keith and her son and daughter-in-law at the bedside. John cared for Elsie's body after death and attended the funeral a week later. Rachael asked John some questions to help him interpret his own experience of caring for Elsie.

Rachael: *What were your hopes for Elsie?*
John: *I hoped she would get well and go home, as she always did.*
Rachael: *How were your hopes for Elsie related to your ideals of 'good' nursing practice?*
John: *Good nursing helps people to get better. Ideally, Elsie would get well and go home again.*
Rachael: *But Elsie did not go home. Does that make you a 'bad' nurse?*
John: *Oh no, no, of course not. I think what gets me is my reaction. I've never cried at work before in all this time!*
Rachael: *So, are your tears the issue here?*
John: *Well, yes, why did I cry? I've cared for so many other people who are dying and they never got to me like Elsie did.*

Rachael: *What are the sources in your life and work for your ideas and values about crying at work?*

John: *I come from the whole 'boys don't cry' tradition. My father always shook my hand when he greeted me, and even though my mother always encouraged me to show my feelings, I could never really get away from dad's influence. It's not that I don't feel emotion; it's just that I don't usually show it.*

John and Rachael continued their conversation about John's tearful reaction to Elsie's impending death. Rachael assisted John to learn from his practice story by asking him some questions to prompt reflection.

Rachael: *John, what does this story about Elsie tell you about your expectations of yourself?*

John: *I expect myself to act professionally at all times at work.*

Rachael: *And that means?*

John: *Not showing my emotions, I guess.*

Rachael: *And now?*

John: *Now it's not so 'cut and dried'. I don't regret crying for Elsie. I loved her so much and I felt genuine sadness for her. Keith was in tears too, because he heard what Elsie said to me. Even though he didn't want to face it, he knew his beloved grand-mother was dying.*

John and Rachael met one week later and in the meantime John had time to think over their conversation and to enfold other insights into his experience of caring for Elsie.

John: *This reflective practice sure gets you in, doesn't it!*

Rachael: *Yes, what's been happening for you John?*

John: *I've been thinking of what we talked about – not all the time – just every now and then.*

Rachael: *And what have you come up with? What have you learned from this situation?*

John: *I was so surprised by my own tears. I didn't know where they came from. Previously, I lived my work life by the thought that a good nurse is a good man, and a good man does not cry. Now, I am not so sure.*

John shared his insights into himself and his practice. Rachael listened intently, nodding her head in assent most of the time, saying nothing. John had come to his own insights and all Rachael did, as his critical friend, was to listen quietly and ask a question here and there.

Rachael: *So John, do you think that your story about Elsie changes your awareness about the ways you communicate at work?*

John: *Definitely. I'm not about to start crying all over the place,*

> *because that is not what it's about for me. I'm coming to understand that I can be a professional and still be able to show my emotions now and then, when they are genuinely from the heart. Maybe that's the best thing I ever did for Elsie – to show her how much I cared for her, had grown to love her, in fact. Getting close to Elsie made me vulnerable, because when she died I felt I had lost a grandmother. But, if I had it all to do over again, I'd still get to know Elsie and risk closeness, in favour of being detached and never really to get to know her as a friend.*

Author's reflection

When I wrote the second edition of this book, I realized that I had evolved a reflective process that could be demonstrated in a model. I love playing with words and ideas, so I toyed with various mnemonics and came upon the REFLECT structure. I express it as 'came upon' because it felt like I had stumbled across it in the dark somehow, and it had made its presence known to me from out of the depths of my creative thoughts. It took reflective effort to make the REFLECT mnemonic materialize, but after it was apparent to me, it seemed so simple and easy. I suppose that's the nature of thinking – turning our attention towards something puts it into focus, brings it to light, makes it apparent and we instantly assimilate it as familiar.

In this edition of the book, I wanted to make the model even more accessible, through an abbreviated, easy to recall and use guide. I have worked in clinical and academic arenas and I have noticed that my colleagues and I entertain and apply ideas to our practice activities if we see them as being easy to recall and use and they are ultimately practical and helpful. So, my hope is that the REFLECT model will be personally and professionally applicable and advantageous for you as a reflective practitioner.

Processes have a way of unfolding, but I have noticed that if I can anticipate the phases of the unfolding to some degree, it decreases my anxiety and enhances the outcomes. For example, as a practising midwife, in fear of 'being front and centre' at a birth, I did not catch on at all to the nuances of birthing until I fully understood the processes of labour and delivery. As an intellectual exercise, I tried learning about the mechanics of the movement of the baby from the uterus and through the birth canal, but the textbook was not enough to help me understand and remember the process. It was only in witnessing many actual births, playing with a clinical lab model, and imagining the concerted efforts of the mother, including her uterine contractions, pelvic floor contours and the propulsion of the baby downwards through the birth canal, that I finally *got it* theoretically and could apply it in my midwifery practice. When I was in a position of needing to teach that process to student midwives, I used the natural flow of the process of mother and baby working together to help novices learn what to expect when caring for a woman during labour and delivery.

Another thing I have realized over time in my personal and professional life is to be ready for the unexpected and to be flexible, or 'roll with the punches' as my dad would say, because unusual things can happen which deviate from the 'normal' processes. No amount of application of processes could have prepared me completely for some of the 'curve balls' my personal life and work have thrown at me, but I have taken comfort in knowing that I've had a semblance of a plan in most cases, and that I am me, with all my human foibles, moving on through life as consciously and as attentively as I can at any given moment.

Summary

In this chapter I encouraged you to apply my REFLECT model to your own healthcare practice, so you can compile a portfolio of your own practice stories in order to find trends and patterns in your practice, which can benefit from your attentive consideration. It is my hope that the abbreviated REFLECT guide will help you to develop expertise as a reflective practitioner and that you come to embody a reflective attitude to your life and your work.

Key points

- The Taylor model of reflection uses the mnemonic REFLECT, to represent Readiness, Exercising thought, Following systematic processes, Leaving oneself open to answers, Enfolding insights, Changing awareness and Tenacity in maintaining reflection.
- An abbreviated guide to using the REFLECT model allows you to access and use it easily and comprehensively for reflecting during or after practice.
- The time you take in reflecting may vary from microseconds, to minutes, to hours, according to your circumstances.
- With increasing levels of expertise as a professional and experience as a reflective practitioner, you can embody the REFLECT process and become unaware of your continually engaged reflective attitude.

8 Reflective practice in research and scholarship

Introduction

This chapter provides practical information on how to incorporate reflective practice into research methodologies and scholarship in the form of health-care knowledge. Reflective methods and processes fit well with all qualitative research methodologies, and this chapter identifies possible applications before focusing on specific projects involving action research. The chapter also describes how to foster scholarship by preparing your research findings for conference presentations and journal articles, because research worth doing is worth sharing to improve practice and to extend interdisciplinary knowledge.

Research is important in any human service providing healthcare, because humans require and deserve high-quality management of their health needs. Ideally, healthcare professionals are mindful of the complexity of their practice and they attempt daily to provide safe and effective care based on the latest research evidence. Reflective methods and processes not only guide practice, they can also provide evidence for supporting practice changes.

Scholarship in healthcare professions is generated and validated through scientific means. 'Science' in this sense is *'scientia'*, meaning knowledge in general, not the specific knowledge of an empirical type originating from the scientific method. This means that *scientia* allows for many types of knowledge that contribute equally to the disciplinary content of healthcare professions. Thus, reflective methods and processes in practice provide empirical, interpretive and critical knowledge for scholarship in healthcare.

Incorporating reflective practice into research methodologies

This section reviews foundational research knowledge before connecting research methodologies to reflection. Research attempts to find new and amended knowledge using systematic data collection and analysis approaches. You may need to consult recent research texts in your profession, because this section cannot cover the detailed complexity inherent in healthcare research methods and processes. As a basis for understanding the connections between reflection and research, it is important to review the main types of research, because they make certain assumptions about how knowledge is generated and verified.

Types of research

It is advisable for a beginning researcher to reduce the complexity of research by thinking of it as fitting into three main types: empirico-analytical (quantitative), interpretive (qualitative) and critical (qualitative) (Taylor *et al*. 2006).

Empirico-analytical (quantitative) research uses numbers and statistics as its main investigative tools, to observe and analyse through the scientific method. The scientific method uses rigorous rules for research, to test something over and over again and be consistently accurate (reliability), and to test what it actually intends to test (validity) rather than other things that are there unnoticed (extraneous variables). To achieve this, the scientific method demands objectivity, to eradicate the distorting influences of people, such as their ideas, intentions and emotions (subjectivity), to produce scientific knowledge. The scientific method only asks research questions that can be structured in ways that can be observed and analysed (by empirico-analytical means), and measured by numbers, percentages and statistics (quantified), hence the categorization of empirico-analytical and/or quantitative research. Research areas examined through quantitative research include cause and effect relationships, incidences and percentages of occurrences and trends. Examples of empirico-analytical research methods are randomized controlled trials, experimental designs, surveys and questionnaires. All of these methods require strict attention to detail, and can be found in most quantitative research texts (e.g. Polit *et al*. 2001).

Reflector

Which type of reflection – technical, practical or emancipatory – combines best with quantitative research methods? Why?

Qualitative research can be interpretive or critical (Taylor *et al*. 2006), and uses words and language as its main exploratory tools. Qualitative researchers are interested in questions that involve human consciousness and subjectivity, and they value humans and their experiences in the research process. Qualitative research involves finding out about the changing (relative) nature of knowledge, which is seen to be special and centred in the people, place, time and conditions in which it finds itself (unique and context-dependent). Qualitative research uses thinking that starts from the specific instance and moves to the general pattern of combined instances (inductive), so it 'grows from the ground up' to make larger statements about the nature of the phenomenon being investigated. Rather than starting with a statement of anticipated relationships (hypothesis), qualitative research begins a project with a broad statement of the area of interest, such as: 'This research explores the nature of the client–practitioner relationship'. The measures for ensuring validity in qualitative research involve asking participants and other people if the experience resonates with them. Reliability is often not an issue in qualitative research, as it is based on the idea that knowledge is relative and dependent on all of the features of the people, place, time and other circumstances (context) of the setting. People are valued as sources of information and their expressions of their personal awareness (subjectivity) are valued as being integral to the meaning that comes out of the research. Qualitative research makes no claims to generate knowledge that can be confirmed as certain (absolute) or even predictive.

Reflector

Which type of reflection – technical, practical or emancipatory – combines best with interpretive qualitative research methods? Why?

Interpretive qualitative research aims mainly to generate meaning, that is, to explain and describe, in order to make sense of phenomena of interest. Examples of interpretive qualitative research include historical methods, grounded theory, phenomenology and ethnography. Qualitative critical research also generates meaning and aims openly to bring about change in the status quo. Examples of qualitative critical research include action research, critical ethnography, feminist research and discourse analysis. Qualitative interpretive and critical research have many similarities, but they differ in terms of their intention to bring about social and political change. By working collaboratively with participants as co-researchers to systematically address research problems, qualitative researchers try to find answers and use them to bring about change. Further details on these and other qualitative interpretive and critical research approaches can be found in Streubert *et al.* (2003) and Taylor *et al.* (2006), or any research text relevant to your healthcare profession.

Reflector

Which type of reflection – technical, practical or emancipatory – combines best with critical qualitative research methods? Why?

It becomes immediately obvious from the preceding overview of foundational ideas that qualitative research fits best with reflection, as both are concerned with the description of human experience for the possibilities of increased understanding, raised awareness and change. Reflective processes may be the main framework for the project, or they may be integrated into other research approaches.

Possible applications of reflection in research

Reflective processes may be used solely as the research approach, or they may be integrated into other research approaches. This section describes both options, to open up the potential for creative reflective processes in research.

The reflective research approach

A research project may use reflective methods and processes solely as its organizing and procedural framework. This is because reflective approaches assume certain principles of knowledge generation and validation that fit well with the qualitative research paradigm. The validation for this position has been provided already in this chapter. Briefly, reflective practice generates objective (through technical reflection) or subjective (through practical and emancipatory reflection), context-dependent, relative knowledge that resonates as 'truth' for the individual and for other people who recognize similar experiences. The value of reflective knowledge of an interpretive or critical form is raised awareness, insight and potential for change and improvement.

The forms of reflection described in this book can be used as data collection methods in research projects. For example, a project examining the effectiveness of a clinical procedure could use technical reflective processes to facilitate critical thinking and problem-solving. The information gained through individual or collective discussions using objective argumentation is data. These processes could be used alone or in combination with other quantitative methods, such as experiments and structured observation. Research participants could keep reflective journals or use the questions posed by technical reflection as a stimulus for group discussion. The aim of research using technical reflection would be to satisfy the need for rational adaptations to work procedures and to maintain evidence-based practice.

Practical reflection may be used in any project which intends to explore the meaning of phenomena in healthcare. For example, a project may explore the meaning of illness as it is experienced. In this case, practical reflection could be encouraged in research participants by asking them to tell a story about the experience of their illness. The questions posed in the reflective process could facilitate the telling of the story to ensure that a rich description is achieved. Alternatively, the researcher or research team could keep reflective logs about their experiences of providing care for people.

Emancipatory reflection fits well with critical research, which aims to expose power relations and change the dominant forces constraining health-care professionals' practice. For example, a group of occupational therapists could form an action research group and work collaboratively to bring about changes in their practice according to what matters most to them. This might mean that each person keeps a reflective log, parts of which are shared in the group to assist in deciding on the direction of the project. The group would work together to assess clinical problems and to suggest and trial strategies for change.

A reflective research approach can be used for projects based solely on the assumptions, methods and processes of reflection. As stated previously, the epistemological assumptions of reflection are that knowledge is partially objective or subjective, context-dependent and relative, making no claim as absolute or certain 'truth', but rather as socially constructed representations of 'truth' that provide tentative answers to issues and problems and to 'useful for now' descriptions of meaning and experience.

There is no 'correct' or 'best' reflective research method. Even so, taking the types of reflection in this book as examples, it is possible to construct a creative method to undertake research. The basic eight steps in the method are to: identify the issue/problem/phenomenon for reflection; decide on the reflective method; clarify its intent; plan the stages in a research proposal; follow the method and use the process; generate insights, institute changes and improvements and continue to reflect on outcomes; report on outcomes; and use the outcomes in practice as evidence.

Step 1: identify the issue/problem/phenomenon for reflection
Practice is a rich ground in which to find puzzles to be solved. Issues and problems can be in relation to the wider health environment – for example, research questions can be raised about governmental structures and processes for health, legal and ethical guidelines for healthcare and the organizational structures and systems in which you work. Research questions can also be raised about your local professional context, such as the department, ward or unit in which you work. The specific nature of the research questions will depend on the issues you locate there, for example, research questions could be about policies and procedures, interpersonal relationships, and/or power plays.

Reflector
Turn to Chapter 1 and review the issues often faced by professionals in your healthcare service. Are any of these issues familiar to you? Choose one and write two research questions in relation to it. This will be the issue you will work on, in order to follow a reflective research process. Write it down as Step 1.

Step 2: decide on the reflective method

In this step you choose the type of reflection that best suits the exploration of your clinical issue. Given that this book sets out three types of reflection, use one of them as the basis for demonstrating this approach to reflective research. Is your issue about policies and procedures, interpersonal relationships or politics at work? Is it a combination of all or some of these? When you make this decision, remember that this book describes technical reflection for policy and procedural issues; practical reflection for interpersonal communication issues; and emancipatory reflection for issues involving unequal power balances.

Reflector

Decide on a reflective method to suit the issue you chose in Step 1. Write it down under the issue as Step 2.

Step 3: clarify the intent of the reflective method

To ensure that the method fits your clinical issue, clarify the intent of the specific type of reflection you are thinking of using in your research. For example, you'll remember that technical reflection offers you the objective means to observe and analyse work procedures through scientific reasoning, because it has an interest in instrumental action. Practical reflection will help you to understand the interpersonal basis of human experiences and offer you the potential for creating new knowledge, because it has an interpretive intent. Emancipatory reflection will give you a method for making a radical critique of the constraining forces and power influences within your work setting, because it has transformative action as its primary concern.

Reflector

What is the intent of the reflective method you have chosen? Is one method enough, or do you need to combine it with one or two other types of reflection to research this issue effectively? Write a sentence or sentences that clarify the intent of the reflective methods you have chosen as Step 3.

Step 4: plan the stages in a research proposal

This step follows the usual stages in any research proposal, that is, the research title, significance, aims, objectives, research questions, background, literature and methodology, and plans for the data collection, analysis, interpretation and dissemination. A timeline and budget may also be necessary. The following description is brief and intended only as an indicator of your need to do further reading (e.g. Polit *et al.* 2001; Streubert *et al.* 2003; Taylor *et al.* 2006), or seek expert advice, if you have not undertaken research previously.

Significance
The significance of the research is the usefulness of the project and it answers the implicit question: why is this research necessary?

Aims and objectives
Aims are overall intentions and objectives are specific subsets of the intentions.

Research questions
Specific questions related to the research objectives are posed at this point. These indicate the problem focus you are taking in the research.

Background
Sometimes a background statement precedes the literature review, to set the context for how the ideas for the research came into being. It serves the purpose of showing the researcher's interest in the project.

Literature review
The aim of a literature review is to locate the information that is available in peer-reviewed journals and books relating as closely as possible to the aims and objectives of your proposed project. This is done in order to shed light on what is already known about your topic of interest, and/or even to decide whether a new project on the topic is necessary. For example, relative lack of information shows that the project is needed, but finding literature relating to many projects of a high standard, all discovering the same ideas, means that the area is well researched and that it most probably does not need further work presently. Research that is similar to, yet different from, the aims and objectives of your research can also be used, to show how other researchers have tackled parallel research questions. Undertaking a critically focused literature review takes practice, and texts are available to help you in your healthcare profession. The main objectives are to locate, analyse and critique relevant literature in terms of its methods, processes and findings, in order to locate strengths and weaknesses in previous projects and thus bring a clearer focus to your proposed project. The length of a literature review varies according to its purposes. Whereas a literature review in a thesis may stretch to thousands of words, a literature review in a research proposal may be only one page or within the limit of the funding body or ethics committee. The references may be included immediately after the literature review, or appear in an appendix attached to the proposal.

Methodology
Methodology refers to the theoretical assumptions underlying the choice of methods. This means that in the proposal under the word 'methodology' there

will be a short description of the theoretical tradition informing the project, in this case, reflective practice and the particular theories informing this research.

Data collection

Full ethical clearance processes precede the commencement of any project involving human participants. The proposal includes the number of participants and access arrangements. It may be necessary to provide a rationale for the number of participants, especially if the proposal is likely to be judged against quantitative criteria of large sample sizes. Ethics committee members may not be aware of the assumptions of the nature of knowledge generated and validated through qualitative research. The extent to which you produce a strongly referenced rationale will depend on the likelihood of it being needed. You might also need to justify your 'sampling' methods, that is, how you will go about accessing the participants.

Be sure to include information on what data you will collect and how you will collect them. Provide examples of the reflective strategies you will use (see Chapter 2). If you are conducting interviews or facilitating discussion, list the questions you intend to ask, even if they are broad guidelines for stimulating conversations.

Data analysis and interpretation

The proposal must set out clearly the methods for sorting (analysing) and making sense of (interpreting) of the data. This is the main way the project will be judged as trustworthy when completed. Therefore, the proposal should be very clear about what you intend to do in order to analyse and interpret the data, so that the people judging the merits of the proposal can consider whether your plans for this phase are reasonable in relation to the rest of the project.

Dissemination of findings

The proposal should contain a plan for the dissemination of findings. This will show that you are aware that the research will be rendered meaningless if the results are not shared with the people who may benefit from them.

The project time frame

The proposal needs to show that you are organized time-wise and that you have allowed enough time to complete the project within the prescribed period. The funding body and/or your organization will want to know what you are going to do, and when, so that they can be assured that the project will be completed on time.

Budget

If you are applying for a research grant to assist you in completing your research, you will need to give careful consideration to the costs involved.

Most grant bodies require a detailed budget, outlining costs for the research personnel (research assistants, desktop publishers, clerical assistance and so on); equipment (computer data analysis system, audiotapes and so on); travel at X pence per mile and other costs, such as photocopying, mailing and so on. The grant application will make it clear what they will or will not fund, so be sure to read their information carefully. Funding bodies want to know about each item of research expenditure in your budget, to satisfy themselves that the money is justified and you will use it prudently.

Reflector

Use the stages in writing a reflective research proposal in Step 4 to outline briefly your proposed research, as projected already in Steps 1 to 3 of this section.

Step 5: follow the method and use the process

Bearing in mind the statements you have made already in the research proposal you projected in Step 4, review the specific type(s) of reflection you have chosen to research your clinical issue. You may need to merge some or all of the three processes (see Chapters 4, 5 and 6), depending on the complexity of the research issue and the nature of your research questions. This is the time to undertake the research, assuming you have gained ethical clearance and you are ready to proceed with confidence, as an individual or team member researcher, or with research supervision as a student in a research programme.

Reflector

Compile the complete proposal, to include the actual reflective process questions you will be using. Before proceeding, ensure that you have ethical clearance, and that you are competent to conduct research, or you have research supervision from an experienced researcher.

Step 6: generate insights, institute changes and improvements and continue to reflect on outcomes

In this part of the research, you start to generate insights and make changes and improvements, depending on your research aims and objectives and the processes you have chosen to fulfil them. Document these events carefully, in accordance with participants' accounts of their experiences for practical and emancipatory reflection, and/or in accordance with the scientific reasoning that develops in the case of technical reflection. Reflect on the outcomes, especially on the extent to which the research aims and objectives have been achieved and what further research may be necessary, to extend or more adequately explore other clinical issues.

Reflector

In relation to the research issue you have been exploring in this section, what insights have you gained, and what practice changes and improvements have you made? Have you achieved the research aims and objectives? Is further research necessary?

Step 7: report on outcomes

In this step you prepare to disseminate your research findings. You will find information in this chapter about giving a professional conference presentation and preparing an article for a refereed journal. If you need further help, seek the advice of an expert researcher or academic, who may be willing to assist you in the process.

Reflector

How will you disseminate your research findings? Use the information in this chapter to assist you to begin the first draft of a conference paper and/or a refereed journal article. If you are new to either process, take your first draft to a researcher or academic, who may be willing to assist you further.

Step 8: use in practice as evidence

In this step you explore the possibility of using your research findings in practice. This may happen through the adaptation of existing policies and procedures in your workplace, or you may decide to submit your work to an organization responsible for validating guidelines for evidence-based practice, for example, the Johanna Briggs Institute in Australia.

Reflector

What are your plans for changing practice by using your research as evidence? Consider how your research may be used as a practical guide to practice, based on its validity as evidence for clinical improvement.

Summary

This section described the basic eight steps in the reflective research method. Research knowledge and skills take time to amass, so if you are new to research you may need guidance beyond this section to prepare you to research competently. If you are ready to undertake research, consider using a reflective research approach based entirely on reflective processes, as described in this section.

Reflective processes in other research approaches

Reflective processes can be used in conjunction with other research approaches, for example quantitative (technical reflection), qualitative (practical and emancipatory reflection) or mixed methods of quantitative and qualitative research (technical reflection, plus one or two other types of reflection used in this book). There is no prescription as to how these approaches might be used, as it is up to the researcher to make those choices, based on the fit of the approach to the research aims and objectives. Of course, any approach to reflective practice can be used within a research project if it adds richness to the data, not just the types described in this book. Other reflective processes in research approaches have been admirably demonstrated (e.g. Freshwater 1999a, 1999b; Handcock 1999; Johns 2000, 2003; Glaze 2001). Even so, for ease of reference and to demonstrate their value, the types of reflection described in this book will be used as examples for how reflective practice can be used in other research approaches.

For example, a quantitative project using a survey or questionnaire might also use the technical reflection process in a focus group to develop scientific reasoning to support or oppose the continuation of a clinical policy or procedure. A qualitative interpretive research approach using ethnography might also include participants' journals, in which descriptions of the research context are written for later analysis and interpretation, thus adding richness to the description of the culture being studied. The practical reflection process may also be used to explore communicative aspects of the culture of interest. A qualitative critical research approach using action research based on critical theory may use the action research cycles, with a special emphasis on reflection (as demonstrated in the next section). The emancipatory research process could be used in any form of critical research that intends to question the status quo and bring about change in people and organizations.

Researchers may use reflective journaling in any project they are undertaking, as a means of demonstrating rigour or trustworthiness, through documenting the detailed life of the project, and the researcher's and target audience's responses to the process and the findings.

Research students enrolled in research programmes may use reflective processes in the design of their projects. They may also keep a reflective account of their experience as a research student, of the project itself, of the learning that comes about through supervisory meetings, their reactions to literature, and any insights along the way that add richness to the research.

Table 8.1 gives some ideas about how reflective processes may be used in research approaches. The list is to demonstrate possibilities; it is not a prescription, nor is it exhaustive. The possibilities are many, so be creative in deciding how you will use reflective processes in your research.

Table 8.1 Possibilities for using reflective processes in research projects

Paradigm	Methodology	Type of reflection	Processes	Strategies
Quantitative	Empirico-analytical	Technical	Scientific reasoning	Focus groups Committees Consumer groups
Qualitative interpretive	Historical research (oral history, autobiographies)	Practical	Experiencing, interpreting, learning	Journal Audiotape Videotape Photography
	Ethnography	Practical	Experiencing, interpreting, learning	Journal Audiotape Painting Drawing Photography
	Phenomenology	Practical	Experiencing, interpreting, learning	Journal Audiotape Videotape Painting Drawing Photography
Qualitative critical	Critical ethnography	Emancipatory	Constructing, confronting, deconstructing, reconstructing	Journal Group work Audiotape Videotape Painting Drawing Photography
	Feminisms	Emancipatory	Constructing, confronting, deconstructing, reconstructing	Journal Group work Audiotape Videotape Painting Drawing Photography Dancing Poetry Montage
	Action research	Emancipatory	Constructing, confronting, deconstructing, reconstructing	Journal Group work Audiotape Videotape Painting Drawing Photography Dancing Poetry Montage

Research involving reflection and action research

This section describes how reflection and action research combine to create an effective collaborative qualitative research approach for identifying and transforming clinical issues. Action research is described and a research approach is outlined that applies the ideas of reflection and action research into a transformative process. Two nursing research projects exemplify the effectiveness of reflection and action research.

Nursing has used reflective processes for some time to improve practice (Taylor 2000; Thorpe and Barsky 2001; Stickley and Freshwater 2002; Johns 2003), clinical supervision (Todd and Freshwater 1999; Heath and Freshwater 2000; Gilbert 2001), education (Freshwater 1999a, 1999b; Johns 2000; Platzer *et al.* 2000a) and research (Freshwater 2001; Taylor 2001, 2002a, 2002b). Midwifery is also a rich source of reflection and midwives have been encouraged to use reflective processes to inform and improve their practice (Taylor 2002a, 2002b). In any healthcare profession involving complex practices in terms of knowledge, skills and human connection, there are many opportunities for using reflection and action research as a collaborative research approach. Reflection is described in detail in this book, so I now introduce action research to demonstrate its synergies with reflective practice.

Action research grew out of World War II (Chein *et al.* 1948) and had a social change agenda. Kurt Lewin (1946) first used the term 'action research' and in the mid-1940s used a group research process for community projects in postwar America. Lewin's work is the basis of contemporary versions of action research, including those forwarded by Australian educationalists such as Carr and Kemmis (1984). Action research goes to the site of the concern or practice, and works with the people there as co-researchers, to generate solutions to the problems with which they are keen to deal.

Action research involves a four-stage process of collectively planning, acting, observing and reflecting (Dick 1995; Stringer 1996). Each phase leads to another cycle of action, in which the plan is revised, and further acting, observing and reflecting is undertaken systematically, to work towards solutions to problems of a technical, practical or emancipatory nature (Kemmis and McTaggart 1988; Taylor 2000). The planning and acting phases may include any appropriate methods of gathering and analysing data, such as participant observation, reflective journaling, surveys, focus groups and interviews. Cycles of action research lead to further foci and co-researchers can keep an action research approach to their work for as long as they choose, to find solutions to their practice problems.

Nurses have been using action research successfully in a variety of settings with differing thematic concerns (e.g. Chenoweth and Kilstoff 1998; Keatinge *et al.* 2000; Koch *et al.* 2000). Midwives have also been using action research to assist them in improving their practice (Deery and Kirkham 2000; Barrett 2001; Munroe *et al.* 2002) and education systems (Fraser 2000; McMorland and Piggott-Irvine 2000).

Combining reflection and action research

Reflective processes and action research combine well to create an effective collaborative qualitative research approach for identifying and transforming clinical issues, because reflection is part of the action research method of planning, assessing, observing and reflecting. Reflection is drawn out especially in this combined approach of collaborative research, because this distinction gives more importance to the role of reflective processes in helping practitioners to make sense of their practice and to bring sustained improvements to it. This section provides a step-by-step approach to facilitating an action research and reflection group.

Facilitating an action research and reflection group

You can set up an action research and reflection group where you work, and it can stay together for as long as you all have practice issues to research collaboratively. Follow these 13 easy steps.

Step 1: find enough healthcare professionals to form a research group
Two or more people comprise a group, so you do not have to seek large numbers of participants when you set up a research group.

Step 2: ensure the healthcare professionals are ready to make a commitment to the research group
Your colleagues will need to commit to working together through their practice issues, so they will need to meet regularly, for as often and as long as they need to work through the research systematically and to the point at which it offers practice insights and improvements. For this to happen, the healthcare professionals will also need to commit to reflecting on their practice and sharing their thoughts with the group.

Step 3: decide on a venue and a regular meeting day and time
It does not matter where you meet, but it must be a venue that allows privacy so that co-researchers can speak openly and confidentially. There may be a quiet room set aside in your organization for employees, or you may decide to meet in a private home. Decide on a regular day and time, for example, every Friday from 2.30 to 3.30 p.m. for one hour. The specifics of this decision will depend on agreement by the healthcare professionals involved.

Step 4: write a brief research proposal

Write a brief proposal of what it is you are going to do, why, when, how and with whom. The essentials of a proposal include the project's title, background, aims, objectives, data collection and analysis methods, timeline, budget and plans for dissemination (as described previously). Specifics of this process can be found in research texts relevant to your healthcare profession. Keep the proposal succinct and in easy to read language, because it is a guide for the group as well as for any other interested audiences, such as a funding body or an ethics committee. Enlist the help of another healthcare professional from your proposed research group in preparing the proposal, or this first writing step could be a collaborative project for the entire group before you start the action research and reflection.

Step 5: check on ethics approval processes in your organization

Because you are undertaking research with other human participants, you may need ethics approval. Check with the ethics committee in your organization what is required for your submission to them. Write in clear, non-jargonistic language and enlist the help of another healthcare professional from your proposed research group in preparing the ethics submission. Alternatively, the ethics approval and proposal writing process could be a collaborative project for the entire group. If you need further help, refer to a relevant research text.

Step 6: get the project under way and decide on who facilitates meetings

When you have the necessary ethics approval you can begin the action research and reflection group meetings, focusing on the methods and processes to get the project under way. Decide if you will have one facilitator for every meeting, or if you will use a 'rotating chair' system, in which everyone takes a turn at guiding the agenda of the regular meetings. You may decide to keep minutes of meetings as a successive account of the research process and for information that can be included in the research report for dissemination.

Step 7: share the business of the first two meetings

At its inception, there are some important foundational processes through which the group must work together. The areas to be discussed openly include group processes, and shared understandings of action research and reflective processes. Group processes are decided by listening to what each healthcare professional wants from the group in terms of how they will work together. For example, they may say that they want to be able to speak openly, with trust and confidentiality, and that nothing discussed in the group will be open to public discussion and so on. So that everyone understands the fundamental ideas in action research and reflection, ensure each healthcare professional reads this chapter and any other useful resources, and shares in group discussion their understanding of these basic tenets and how they relate to researching their practice.

Step 8: share the first reflective task

Take as many meetings as you need to work through the first reflective task. It is important to begin here, because it gives participants in the research group confidence in writing or recording their reflections and sharing them in the group. Use the guide in this book (see Chapter 2) as the first reflective practice writing task. It is an opportunity for participants to reflect on their own personal, social and historical contexts, so that they can consider the values and 'rules for living' that have contributed to how they now live and practise. When each participant shares his or her responses, it is important that the other co-researchers listen attentively and non-judgementally. This may be the first trusting contribution co-researchers make to the group, so it is important to respect and honour the responses for the insights they give into the personal–professional life of the participant.

Step 9: share the practice stories

The next part of the research is to begin to reflect on present or past practice stories. The reason for doing this is to identify a common theme ('thematic concern', in action research language) through which to work collaboratively. Take as many meetings as you need to work through the first part of the process, because it is important that participants share at least two practice stories with the group. Use the guides in this book (Chapters 4, 5 and 6) to reflect on practice stories. The guides assist you to make a critical analysis of an incident at work, according to whether it is primarily of a work procedure, communication or power nature, or any combination of these issues. Keep in mind that the aim of the research group is to locate issues of interest to participants in order to raise awareness and change practice through action research and reflective processes. After the group has worked together for a while, decide on issues that are common to everyone (thematic concerns) and use an action research approach to work through them.

When each participant shares her or his practice stories, it is again important that the other co-researchers listen attentively and non-judgementally. It is not usually a part of healthcare culture to speak openly about practice stories that did not go well, so be careful to honour the stories, allowing the storyteller to find his or her own insights. Co-researching participants may act as critical friends (see Chapter 2) by asking question for a fuller description, or to encourage a wider exploration of the issue, but they should not offer easy solutions, because it is best to avoid an early foreclosure on possibilities.

Step 10: identify the thematic concern(s)

Keep summary notes of each story and devise a method for analysing their contents. For example, construct a grid with four columns, including 1) story summary, 2) the issue(s), 3) the healthcare professional's feelings about the issue(s), 4) how the issue(s) came about. The second column will be most useful in locating the issues to find some thematic concerns common to each participant. For example, the analysis may show that participants have issues relating to relationships, such as with other healthcare professionals, patients, relatives and so on. The third column will identify the emotions and feelings participants experience in day-to-day practice, which are at the foundation of their perceptions of their practice. The fourth column will locate the various sources of participants' work issues, which affect the ways in which they negotiate their practice conditions. Spend some time discussing the analysis of the stories, with particular interest in the practice issues that are identified. See if there are any issues that come up consistently in the stories. Decide on an issue to research together using an action research and reflection process. If there are several thematic concerns and enough participants in the group to work on them effectively, it is possible to work on many issues at the same time.

Step 11: generate the action plan and begin the action research cycles

This step of the research lasts as long as it takes for the group to reach satisfactory outcomes. The group is now at the point where they are ready to 'do' action research. The main phases of action research are: Plan, Act, Observe, Reflect (PAOR). Participants begin with a thematic concern (common to enough of them to matter) and move through a series of cycles of PAOR until they feel that the issue is solved/acknowledged/challenged or whatever they hope to achieve in relation to it. This is how it works.

Planning

- The group projects a plan in relation to the thematic concern.
- The plan must be flexible to allow for unforeseen effects and constraints.
- The action prescribed by the plan must take account of the social risks involved and recognize the material and political constraints in the situation.
- The plan allows participants to go beyond their present constraints to empower them to act more effectively in the situation.
- The group plans by collaborating openly and honestly with one another and by analysing and improving their understanding of the situation.

Here are some practical notes for creating an action plan. Construct a grid with three columns, including 1) the thematic concern, 2) the source(s) of the thematic concern, and 3) what can be done about it? The second column will be most useful in locating the sources of the thematic concerns, because they are the work aspects that need some adjustment. For example, if a source of the thematic concern is due to economic constraints, a strategy for the action plan may involve inviting a person 'holding the purse strings' to meet with the group to discuss the concern. If the source of a concern is cultural, in its broadest sense of the way people relate to one another, the focus will be on interpersonal relationships. For example, relationships become defined over time in certain ways, and if there are power imbalances, such as one person exerting 'power over' another person, a strategy may be to observe inter-personal interactions at work in order to examine, and work towards changing, the cultural foundations of these relationships.

When the group is discussing the strategies for the action plan, keep in mind the basic principles listed previously. It is very important to maximize the potential for the success of the action plan by making the strategies within it reasonable for managing the risks and ensuring the best possible outcomes. The action plan will be instituted in healthcare practice and the results of the changed approach to the thematic concern will be noted, through continued PAOR. The action plan will undergo revision until it achieves positive changes in successfully managing the identified thematic concern in practice.

Acting

- The group makes a critically informed, careful and thoughtful variation to practice by putting their plan into action.
- As the strategies in the action plan may be potentially risky, participants need to be flexible and open to change in the light of the real-time situation.
- Acting may involve material, social and political struggle towards improvement and negotiation, and compromise may be necessary.
- Participants may need to be content with modest gains that gradually get bigger based on previous gains (in other words, they may not always be able to 'fix things' the first time).

Observing

- This phase is what makes action research. It involves documenting the effects of critically informed action.
- Participants use their powers of observation and stay responsive, open-eyed and open-minded to see how the plan of action is working.
- Participants record their observations in their journal or by whatever additional means they decide.

- Participants observe the action, the effects of the action (intended and unintended), the circumstances and constraints of the action, and any other issues that may arise.

Reflecting

- Reflection recalls action as it has been recorded in the observation, but it is active in making sense of processes, problems, issues and constraints that may manifest in the strategic action.
- Reflection is aided by group discussion in research meetings so participants can reconstruct the meaning of the social situation and revise the plan if necessary.
- Reflection asks participants to evaluate the effects and the issues and to suggest ways of proceeding.
- Reflection allows reconnaissance for further action research cycles as necessary. Participants keep using the action plan in daily practice until they know they have achieved their aims (plans) relating to the specific issues they raised.

Step 12: write a research report

Use the same structure suggested for the research proposal to write the research report. The front page provides the authors' names (in alphabetical order), positions and qualifications, and the research abstract. The main headings and subheadings under which to write are the title, significance, aims, objectives, research questions, background, literature review, data collection, analysis and interpretation methods and processes, and discussion and conclusions.

The report reiterates much of the information of the proposed research, but in the past tense, because the aim of the report is to give a description of the past events within the project. The report will be written according to the requirements of its target audience – for example, if it is for a funding body the report may be quite lengthy and detailed, but if it is for local dissemination only, it may be short and with just enough detail to describe the project effectively. If you need further help, refer to a relevant research text.

Step 13: disseminate the findings

The final step of the process is to disseminate the research findings, so that the action research and reflection process not only helps the participants but also other people with whom it resonates. If participants in the group have not had previous professional publication and presentation experience, ask for the help of people who have, and invite them to assist the group in the final stage. Alternatively, the group could learn the processes needed by working together through information for contributors supplied by journals and conference committees, ensuring a fair division of labour throughout the learning process. Practical advice is also given in this chapter.

Research projects using reflection and action research

The methods and processes described in the previous section were developed during projects I facilitated with nurses (Taylor 2001; Taylor *et al.* 2002).

The first project (Taylor 2001) was entitled: 'Identifying and transforming dysfunctional nurse-nurse relationships through reflective practice and action research'. It aimed to facilitate reflective practice processes in experienced registered nurses, in order to: raise critical awareness of practice problems; work systematically through problem-solving processes to uncover constraints; and improve the quality of care given by nurses in the light of the identified constraints and possibilities. Twelve experienced female registered nurses working in a large Australian rural hospital shared their experiences of nursing during three action research cycles. A thematic concern of dysfunctional nurse–nurse relationships was identified, as evidenced by bullying and horizontal violence. The negotiated action plan was put into place and co-researchers reported varying degrees of success in attempting to improve nurse–nurse relationships. This project confirmed the necessity for reflective practice and continued collaborative research processes in the workplace to bring about a cultural change within nurses' collectives and in the places in which they work which weigh against mutual respect and cooperation in nurse–nurse relationships.

The second project (Taylor *et al.* 2002) was entitled: 'Exploring idealism in palliative nursing care through reflective practice and action research'. This project also used a combination of action research and reflective practice processes. Six experienced registered nurses identified their tendency towards idealism in their palliative nursing practice, which they defined as the tendency to expect to be 100 per cent effective all of the time in their work. Participants collaborated in generating and evaluating an action plan to recognize and manage the negative effects of idealism in their work expectations and behaviours. Participants expressed positive changes in their practice, based on adjusting their responses to their idealistic tendencies towards perfectionism.

Both projects gave nurses a regular forum in which to discuss their reflections on practice and to generate an action plan to bring about change. The benefits of action research and reflection are that there are immediate, practical outcomes for participants, because they can share their experiences with peers, work together on thematic concerns and bring about local changes in their practice. Thus, co-researchers experience participatory research, while developing their reflective skills, and in this sense the research offers them personal and professional gains in lifelong appreciation of their participation.

Summary

This section gave step-by-step guidance in facilitating an action research and reflection group and described two projects which used the approach successfully. Once you are under way with a project of your own, you will find that the group's enthusiasm will keep the process alive and that you will go from one thematic concern to another, solving clinical issues through action research and reflection.

Fostering scholarship

Scholarship in healthcare professions is generated through sharing interdisciplinary knowledge and skills, and the main modes of dissemination are professional conference presentations and publications. This section outlines how to go about preparing your research findings for dissemination.

Author's reflection

My work as an academic meant that I had to present my research and scholarship at professional seminars and conferences, and after many years of teaching and public speaking, it did not really present any worries for me. However, it wasn't always 'plain sailing'. Speaking up in front of other people began in my family, where I was encouraged to share stories. However, my excited, 'all over the place' sharing with my family of what happened on a school camp or a Sunday School picnic was not the speaking style I needed in later life, when making serious presentations to my work peers, although it grounded me in having confidence in speaking.

My teaching career began during my studies in nurse education. I was to do my 'prac teaching' at a women's hospital in Sydney, Australia. Up until that time, I had undertaken informal teaching roles in practice situations, for example, in a rural hospital where I worked as a registered nurse and midwife, I mentored newly graduated midwives in the practicalities of caring for a woman in labour and delivery. My first teaching engagement was a very different scenario though, complete with a room of 20 or so student midwives, eager to understand complex facts, such as the physiology of labour and foetal circulation.

On my first day of prac teaching, I had to travel by bus along a busy arterial road from way out in the suburbs to the centre of the city. Even allowing copious time, I still found myself running the last few blocks to the midwifery training school, where I was greeted by the principal teacher, who had been looking anxiously out of a side door for my arrival. After a hurried greeting, I was ushered into a classroom, with students seated in a semicircle, attending to a staff member who was speaking at the time I entered. Not wishing to interrupt her, I walked behind the arc of students, not seeing some educational posters hanging from a ledge at shoulder height around the wall. The staff member at the front announced me, and sensing that I was 'on', I bustled around the back of the semicircle, knocking most of the posters off the wall as I went. My quiet unobtrusive entrance had been anything but that, leaving me red-faced and with a real urge to laugh out loud. I still smile when I see myself, feeling so new and frightened, yet trying to remain 'professional'. If I could revisit that scenario again, with the experience I have now, I would feel quite fine about laughing out loud, turning my embarrassment into humour.

The years rolled by and I taught in hospital schools of nursing, until I moved into the tertiary sector with nursing education in the 1980s. I had plenty of practice in teaching nurses and midwives preparing for registration and I revelled in the challenges and delights of classroom and clinical teaching. I was studying by distance learning for a Bachelor of Education at the time, where I was introduced to reflective practice by impressive teachers, such as Stephen Kemmis, John Smyth and Annette Street. When I began work as an academic at Deakin University in 1988, I gained copious experience in presenting my work at conferences, starting as a novice with self-conscious, poorly timed presentations, and gradually developing expertise as an at-ease, articulate speaker with an innate sense of timing. There were many experiences in the stages between novice to expert speaker, and I have attempted in this chapter to distil my learning down to the 'tin tacks' of how to survive and enjoy public speaking at professional conferences.

Learning about teaching and presenting at conferences as I developed as an academic did not mean I became invincible by foreseeing all contingencies that would ensure a 'good' presentation or prevent embarrassment. In fact, 'fancy footwork' was needed at my very last official conference presentation as a full-time academic, when I was a keynote speaker at an international caring conference held in Western Australia. Many luminaries in nursing and caring were there, including my personal favourites, Jean Watson and Dawn Freshwater. I was not a bit nervous as I sat out front waiting to be introduced. I actually wondered what it would take to make me nervous as a speaker at a conference, and I was feeling totally at ease.

The presentation was about the 'Taylor model of reflection' and I was feeling fairly proud of presenting the REFLECT mnemonic to my distinguished and attentive audience. All went well with timing, relating to the audience and so on, until the PowerPoint slide depicting the diagram of the sphere of practice and the meaning of the REFLECT mnemonic. I said with great flourish: 'And this is a diagram of the model' and looked up to the blank screen. The diagram was not there! A quick double take made me realize that salvage was not possible at this point, so in a flash, I joked: 'I can assure you that there is more to the model than that!' The audience erupted in laughter with me and I went on to paint a work picture of the model, with no embarrassment or ill effect from the blank screen where the diagram should have been.

As I write this reflection, I realize that my public teaching and speaking began and ended with potentially embarrassing experiences. I've learned a lot about life and myself since my first day of prac teaching, but probably two of the best things are that I don't have to be perfect or invincible and that it is possible to recover from most near disasters with humour.

Presenting your reflective research at a professional conference

For the uninitiated, the prospect of standing up in front of a group of people and speaking about your experiences and insights may be daunting. Public speaking requires courage to endure the scrutiny of your ideas. This section advises you on how to prepare to present your research or reflective practice experiences, by choosing the gathering, writing the abstract, preparing the paper, and preparing yourself on the day and at the presentation. In conclusion, some thoughts are shared about managing afterwards, in terms of praise and critique, and other outcomes such as conversion of the paper into an article for publication.

Choosing the gathering

When you are choosing the gathering at which to speak, think about the theme of the conference, how your presentation contributes, the potential audience and practical aspects such as your availability and any costs involved. When conference organizers send out their advertising material, they describe the theme of the conference and the subthemes which fit within it. Some conferences have a very specific focus, such as 'Reflective practice as evidence-based practice' while others leave areas open for interpretation, for example, 'Making a difference in practice'.

After reading the advertising material, decide how your presentation would contribute to the conference. You can be creative by making indirect links with conference themes, so don't be deterred by what may appear to be a specific and limited theme. Consider the professional and public mix of the potential audience, and choose a conference at which your presentation will have the most appropriate appeal.

Pay attention to practical aspects. Check the dates and times of the conference to ensure that your diary is free, and that you can cover, or encourage your organization or other agents to sponsor, any costs involved. Submitting an abstract gives the organizers the impression that you are willing and available to be chosen as a conference speaker, and an apparent 'change of mind' on your part may not be received favourably.

Writing the abstract

Unless you are invited as a guest speaker, you will normally need to write an abstract of your proposed presentation. Most organizers provide a space for you to complete an abstract on the conference information sheet, which is returned to them for review and selection procedures. You need to ensure that what you intend to present fits the conference theme and is sufficiently interesting to catch the attention of the selection committee. Many organizers undertake a 'blind review', which means they take the applicant's name and contact details off abstracts and the selection committee judges the merit of the abstract against their selection criteria, rather than in terms of the personal characteristics or reputation of the speaker.

Notice in the guidelines for abstract writing the word limit and any other stylistic features, such as double spacing, and whether it is to be typed and to contain references to literature. Typing should not present a problem by word processing, because you can format the dimensions of the page, type the abstract, make a copy of the computer document, and paste it into the space provided. References are seldom expected in a conference abstract, but if your paper has a particular focus in the literature you will need to cite the work of published authors. You will also need to decide on a title for the paper, and to state clearly your objectives for the session and the general direction of the presentation. It is a good idea to use a selection of the main words in the conference theme within your abstract, to show the organizers that you have considered the relevance of your contribution.

The abstract should represent a commitment to what you present on the day. Conference delegates select their sessions carefully on the basis of the published abstract, and they may be annoyed or disappointed to find the presenter say at the start of the presentation, 'My abstract indicates X, however, today I will be presenting Y'.

Preparing the presentation

You may receive a letter, email or phone call informing you that your abstract has been selected for a conference. Having kept a copy of the abstract and the other conference details, you can refer to them to refresh your memory on your proposed presentation and the conference venue, day and time. The organizers may request a copy of the paper prior to the conference, so that it can be included in the published proceedings. They will give you a timeline for submission and directions for the format, style and form in which to present the paper.

As with all writing tasks, you need to take some time to prepare a plan for the beginning, middle and end of the paper. Feel free to adapt the following approach to suit yourself. If you have a disk copy of the abstract, make a duplicate of the document and use that as the structure for the paper. Use the return key on the computer keyboard to segment out the main ideas of the paper, in the order you have written them. These small segments may become headings or subheadings, but at this point they remind you of where you are going with the presentation. Sometimes the abstract will not reflect all the twists and turns of your talk, so add these areas under appropriate headings, or create a heading to accommodate them. This does not necessarily mean that the paper is different from what you proposed, but that more information has come to light in the period between the abstract submission and acceptance.

Using the headings, write the paper. You don't necessarily have to start at the beginning and finish at the end, even though you have made a plan for the overall paper. Word processors are great for jumping around the text where you fancy, as a thought comes, or a link in the discussion emerges. Try to write according to the 'tone' of the conference. For example, use a casual style of writing and relating to the audience at a highly interactive and experiential conference, or a more formal tone at a conference at which there will be a great deal of serious scholarly debate and the expectation is that you will be clever. If you are not able to judge the tone of the conference, re-read the conference material or contact one of the conference organizers to discuss this with them. Failing that, aim for clarity, midpoint on the 'clever index' and less, rather than more, detail.

How much to write is an important point. It is a sad experience (if the person is about to be stopped by the facilitator) or a frustrating experience (if the person rushes on unabated) to see a nervous presenter galloping through a paper with five minutes to go, having just finished the introduction. With this in mind, practise reading your paper aloud at conference speed to see if it fits well into the time slot allotted to you. With experience you will become adept at timing. I often joke that as a speaker I am like a gas, in that I can expand or contract my talking to fill the available space.

When the paper is ready, keep a copy for yourself to use for the presentation, so that you can write little reminders on it to yourself. For example, make notes such as to thank the organizers for inviting you to speak, or add a bit more information about yourself extra to the introduction, or acknowledge any current major event which may have a bearing on the conference, or honour cultural considerations, such as in acknowledging the indigenous/ traditional owners of the land, or insert a reminder to show an overhead transparency or slide, and so on. Such personalized notes on papers can give you a sense of confidence that you have 'covered all your bases', and you can respond to any unforeseen events as they arise, such as power and equipment failures and people walking in late.

One last hint is to look carefully over the paper and imagine the kinds of questions you might be asked at the end of the presentation. If you have included theoretical concepts or references to scholarly work, be sufficiently conversant with them to be able to answer any questions with relative confidence.

Preparing yourself on the day

Before you leave home on the day of the conference, make a quiet and thorough check of all your papers to ensure that you have all the information you need to locate the venue, and that you have your paper and any audio-visual aids you are using. Keep them in sight on the way to the venue, making sure you have them in your grasp when you leave your form of transport. Plan to arrive at the conference venue in plenty of time for your presentation. This will avert last-minute rushes and heart-stopping situations, such as being caught in city traffic ten minutes before you are due on the podium.

When you arrive, register at the conference desk and be recognized as a speaker. You may be given a special name badge or a coloured ribbon to signify your speaker status. The person facilitating your session will probably be looking for you, so make yourself known so that they can rest assured that you are present and ready. Unless you have a burning need to interact with other people before your presentation, desist from doing this, as it may accelerate your nervousness. Simply ensure that the facilitator has any aids you may be using if you want assistance with them, agree on the signal to activate help, and sit down quietly. If you are well known to many people there and enjoy some 'celebrity status', you may need to find some silent space outside the building, or you could take a slow and gentle walk to a wash room to brush your hair and check on your appearance. A few deep breaths and an internal affirmation or prayer for help may also be useful at this time. Know that you are there to offer your ideas and that they are worthy of being shared.

Giving the presentation

After the introduction, walk to the podium to give your presentation. Watch your footing as you walk and look up and give a smile (if you can) when you reach the podium. Take some time to position your paper on the lectern and look around the room briefly before you begin. This allows you to see the audience as friendly humans, who are there to support you by listening to what you have to say. It is a privilege to have the attention of people. You have prepared for this moment, you feel honoured to be there, so feel confident to allow your presentation to flow, knowing that it is correct in terms of timing and detail.

If you are very new to public speaking, it might help to stand with your feet slightly apart to give you good balance and to lock your knees ever so slightly to keep you upright. All that remains is for you to read the paper as you practised it. Try to look up as much as possible and direct your gaze to people in various parts of the room. As with any communicative episode, this talk will be more interesting if you can use an appropriate tone, pitch and pace, with an occasional smile. If your mouth gets dry, take a drink of water, even if it means stopping to get the facilitator's attention to assist you. If you try to talk with a dry mouth it may aggravate any nervousness already there. Take notice of this sympathetic nervous system reaction, slow down, take a drink, refocus yourself and continue.

As you progress through the paper, be aware of time passing and ensure that you are keeping the pace correct. If you have practised well and there is just enough detail, your only problem on the day may be too much time, because it may be tempting to speak too rapidly. If this is the case, notice how much time you have remaining and slow down 'in flight', so to speak. When the paper is finished, indicate this by saying 'thank you' and wait to see if questions are to be directed to you.

If you are one of many speakers in a session, the facilitator may prefer to wait until the last speaker has finished before offering opportunities for questions. When you are answering a question, consider your response briefly, ensure that you can be heard, and respond as carefully and helpfully as you can. Sometimes people's questions may be longer than your answer, especially if they are preceding their question with background comment. Simply wait, listen and respond directly. If you get a question you cannot answer, respond as honestly as possible, along the lines of 'I have not thought of that. I cannot answer that at the moment', or 'Although you have made an interesting point, it was not my intention to cover that area specifically in this paper/ project'. Remember that you don't have to have all the answers and a gentle deflection of a question may be preferable to bluffing your way recklessly through uncharted theoretical territory.

Managing afterwards

When your talk is over, there will be applause and then you return to your seat in the auditorium, or accompany the other delegates to a refreshments break, or presentations elsewhere. At this point, you will probably encounter further praise or questions from people who remained silent in question time. On other occasions, people will approach you to make connections and some may want to set up networks so that you can keep in touch in relation to some common interests. If you are not accustomed to 'being in the limelight', you may find the attention disconcerting or overwhelming, but you can handle it graciously with a simple 'Thank you'.

If someone is interested in further debate on the content of your paper, you can make a choice about when to attend to his or her request for discussion. Some questions can be answered with a brief reply, while others demand more time to be dealt with adequately. If the discussion has the potential to be protracted, it is a good idea to negotiate a time in which to meet or to exchange contact details. This ensures that you are not deprived of some quiet time after your presentation, or the chance to attend conference sessions in which you are interested.

Another area you might need to consider is the possibility of transforming your presentation into an article for publication. Most conference papers need to be reworked to accommodate the style and tone of individual journals. Check with the conference organizers about copyright if your work has been published in the conference proceedings, otherwise you are at liberty to submit your paper elsewhere. A conference presentation is an important career event, so ensure that you add it to your curriculum vitae.

Reflector

If you have ever presented at a professional conference, what particular aspects were most challenging for you? Why? How will you adjust your next attempt in view of that experience and the hints provided in this section?

Writing a journal article

You may decide that your reflective insights are worth sharing on a broader stage, so you could consider preparing an article for publication. You could write for a local audience, such as in a hospital newsletter, or you could aim for national and international journals, which have non-refereed and refereed sections. You could write alone or in collaboration with a key person, such as your critical friend or colleagues. You could enlist the assistance of a local health studies school, or you could read some books on the subject and do it yourself.

This section gives you some practical advice on how to get started. The first point is to be aware that you are capable of writing for a journal. Don't let self-doubt overtake you. It is compelling to look at other people's articles in journals and think that you cannot attain such standards. Take heart in the knowledge that every author had to start somewhere and go through the experience of submitting work and waiting for feedback. As a former editor of a journal I can assure you that editors and referees will be willing to guide you to publish your article. Take some time preparing for the article, then write, and you may surprise yourself.

Choose a journal

You need to choose a journal which would welcome your reflective practice article. Browse in the healthcare professions journal section of your library and find journals which have the kind of style and content aligning well with reflective practice. Notice the section about information for contributors that is often printed inside front or back covers. This tells you what the editor expects of you in preparing a manuscript for submission. Make a photocopy so that you can study it carefully and use it to plot your way through the task of writing an article. Notice the word limits for each category of articles and the preferred referencing style.

Have a clear focus

It is important to be specific about the direction your article will take. You may have some general ideas at first, which you tease out by 'playing' with a working title, and under that tentative heading, then section off a beginning, middle and end, and list some ideas under each main section to 'fill out' the content. Try to list the ideas in the order of their presentation, in flow of discussion or debate. If your creative thoughts come randomly you can insert ideas anywhere in the general structure of the plan, and move them around until you have a reasonable flow of ideas. When you are clear about the focus of your paper, decide on the actual title and prepare the manuscript according to the journal's guidelines.

Writing a descriptive article

The way of writing differs according to the type of article. For example, if you are writing a descriptive article on your experience of being a reflective practitioner, you will be relating a personal story. If you are writing for a scholarly journal and the article is to be peer reviewed, you will need to demonstrate theoretical prowess and the appropriate use of literature to substantiate your work. As with all writing, the article will need a beginning, middle and end. An introduction presents the theme or point of contention of the paper. A middle part provides the 'guts' or substantive part of the article and will relate the main aspects of the experience. A conclusion usually pulls all the ideas together by making a concise analysis of the event and offering insights for further contemplation.

Writing a research article

If you are writing about a research project which focused on reflection or used it as a method, the usual conventions of preparing a research article apply. If you want to present a synopsis of the entire project, your challenge will be to 'do justice' to the project while keeping to the word limit. You will have to make hard decisions about what to put in and take out of the article, so that the essential features of the project remain intact. Essentially, research reports deal with the project's title, background, aims, objectives, data collection and analysis methods and processes, results, implications and discussion. If you are unsure about the specific content of the essential features of a research report, consult a relevant reference on critique of research.

Checking the drafts

The writing phase will take several drafts. You need to check the manuscript for spelling and grammatical errors, attention to referencing conventions and the layout of headings and subheadings. Ensure that ideas flow between sections and that the discussion and conclusion sections are well substantiated with literature and sound reasoning. It is a good idea to invite the critique of friends and colleagues with experience in reading and writing journal articles. After you have adjusted the manuscript according to their feedback, prepare the copies as specified by the journal's guidelines and add other requirements, such as a title page, contact details and so on. Send it with a covering letter to the editor and await feedback.

Receiving feedback

Refereed journals use a process of peer review to judge the worthiness of your paper against the criteria the journal values in acceptable writing. This means that the editor will remove references to your name and identity and send your paper to at least two people who have expertise in the area the article covers. The editor considers the reviewers' feedback and decides what, if anything, needs to be done to amend the paper before it is ready for publication.

In time, a letter or email will arrive from the editor, informing you whether your article is to be published. Sometimes you will receive a rejection. It is possible that you have misjudged the appropriateness of the journal for the type of article you had written, or that it was simply not 'up to scratch'. As odd as it might seem, rejections may be good experiences for you, for what they can teach you about yourself and your responses to feedback and critique. Although rejection may hurt, realize that it is directed at your writing, not you specifically, and that you can always try again.

A happier message in the editor's letter will be that your article will be published, subject to you making the required changes. Feedback from reviewers will be supplied to assist you in adjusting the manuscript. At this stage, you may consider that there has been a complete misreading of your work (and it can happen!) and you do not want to compromise the article by making changes. You can decide to withhold your work and submit it to another journal. You are under no obligation to inform the editor that you have decided against making the changes as specified. The non-return of your manuscript will signal your lack of further cooperation in the process. You could try to defend your article as written, but the peer review process favours the word of reviewers in judging the merit of scholarly work, even if they 'get it wrong' sometimes. Some editors may negotiate a compromise if they can see the value of what you are arguing, but it is a rare situation that puts the blind review process in question.

Alternatively, the letter may indicate that your article is flawless and ready to publish as is, or it may inform you that the manuscript is not suitable for publication in that particular journal. If you receive notification that it is not suitable for publication, you could resubmit the manuscript elsewhere, after adapting it to another journal's requirements and style. If you want to publish, don't take rejections too much to heart, and don't give up, because 'success begets success'!

Reflector

If you have ever written an article for a professional journal, what particular aspects were most challenging for you? Why? How will you adjust your next attempt in view of that experience and the hints provided in this section?

Summary

This chapter provided practical information on how to incorporate reflective practice into research methodologies and professional scholarship. Reflective methods and processes fit well with all qualitative research methodologies, and this chapter identified possible applications before focusing on specific projects involving action research. The chapter also described how to foster scholarship by preparing your research findings for conference presentations and journal articles. Although it may take some time and work before you feel confident in disseminating research and scholarship contributions to your discipline, don't forget that it can be fun and that confident writing and speaking are within your grasp with practice. They will be even more rewarding if you apply reflective processes to your learning experiences, as you develop your interests in research and scholarship.

Key points

- Reflective methods and processes not only guide practice, they can also provide evidence for supporting practice changes.
- It is advisable for a beginning researcher to reduce the complexity of research by thinking of three main types: empirico-analytical (quantitative), interpretive (qualitative) and critical (qualitative).
- Empirico-analytical (quantitative) research uses numbers and statistics as its main investigative tools, to observe and analyse through the scientific method.
- Qualitative research can be interpretive or critical and it uses words and language as its main exploratory tools.
- Interpretive qualitative research aims mainly to generate meaning, that is, to explain and describe, in order to make sense of phenomena of interest. Examples include historical methods, grounded theory, phenomenology and ethnography.
- Qualitative critical research also generates meaning and aims openly to bring about change. Examples of qualitative critical research include action research, critical ethnography, feminist research and discourse analysis.

- By working collaboratively with participants as co-researchers to systematically address research problems, qualitative researchers try to find answers and use them to bring about change.
- Reflective processes may be used solely as the research approach, or they may be integrated into other research approaches.
- The basic eight steps in the reflective research method are: identify the issue/problem/phenomenon for reflection; decide on the reflective method; clarify its intent; plan the stages in a research proposal; follow the method and use the process; generate insights, institute changes and improvements and continue to reflect on outcomes; report on outcomes; and use the outcomes in practice as evidence.
- Reflective processes can be used in conjunction with other research approaches, and there is no prescription as to how these approaches might be used, as it is up to the researcher to make those choices, based on the fit of the approach to the research aims and objectives.
- Reflective processes and action research combine well to create an effective collaborative qualitative research approach for identifying and transforming clinical issues, because reflection is part of the action research method of **Plan, Act, Observe** and **Reflect** (PAOR).
- The 13 steps to undertake action research and reflection are: find enough healthcare professionals to form a research group; ensure the healthcare professionals are ready to make a commitment; decide on a venue and a regular meeting day and time; write a brief research proposal; check on ethics approval processes in your organization; get the project under way and decide who facilitates meetings; share the business of the first two meetings; share the first reflective task; share the practice stories; identify the thematic concern(s); generate the action plan and begin the action research cycles; write a research report; and disseminate the findings.
- Scholarship in healthcare is generated through sharing interdisciplinary knowledge and skills, and the main modes of dissemination are professional conference presentations and publications.

9   Being human and reflection as a lifelong process

Introduction

Healthcare professions serve humanity. Clients and practitioners are human. Recognizing and sharing our humanity is central to all human healthcare, therefore, this chapter reiterates the importance being human in your profession, while maintaining the high standards of knowledge and skills required to practice safely and authentically.

The maintenance of your reflective practices will require personal and group supports, so that your good intentions materialize into lifelong reflective approaches to your life and work. In this chapter I suggest some ways of maintaining reflective practice by affirming yourself as a reflective practitioner, responding to the critiques, creating a daily habit, seeing things freshly, staying alert to practice, finding support systems, sharing reflection, getting involved in research and embodying reflective practice.

Honouring humanity

In Chapter 3, I described a model of humanness in healthcare, transposed from my PhD research to any healthcare professional. The original qualitative research (Taylor 1988) was with nurses, and its intention was to explore the 'ordinary' everydayness of nurses and patients in a healthcare setting. Because its focus was on nurse–patient relationships and the day-to-day aspects of care, the phenomenon of ordinariness emerged as shared human qualities. Humanness is the core of any relationship with clients in healthcare settings, regardless of the profession of the health carer, thus this model transposes to any healthcare professional who resonates with the idea of honouring humanity in their practice.

If we take a holistic view of human beings, we ascribe to the idea that humans are multidimensional and that they are greater than the sum of their parts – for example, their physical, psychological and spiritual aspects. Taken in its most positive light, humans are spirit-filled beings, united in the extraordinary potential of their ordinary humanity. Like 'fairies in gumboots', humans are greater than they know, as interconnected incarnate beings, with their feet weighted firmly to the ground. Humans are earthed to daily routines and obligations that keep their attention to the apparent emotional polarities of life. In living their daily routines, they may have forgotten something of their spiritual heritage and their interconnectedness with all things, but interpersonal relationships have the potential to remind them every now and then of the beauty and power of their human existence.

Interpersonal relationships are facilitated to some extent through people-oriented healthcare professions, which seek to serve other human beings, and have wonderful opportunities to serve humanity through clinical knowledge and skills and human embodiment. In this sense, being human in healthcare contributes to therapeutic outcomes and honours humanity. The connectedness of being human has the potential to transcend differences between clients and healthcare professionals, to unify them in human relationships that can become in themselves powerful sources of caring and healing. When humanity is honoured in healthcare, clients and professionals have opportunities to recognize one another as humans, through a sensing that acknowledges their shared 'allowingness', 'straightforwardness', 'self-likeness', 'homeliness', 'favourableness', 'intuneness', 'lightheartedness' and 'connectedness' (Taylor 1991).

The shared affinity clients and healthcare professionals can have for each other as humans is not, as might be first thought, a small and inconsequential thing. The ordinariness of the shared affinity of being human can permeate healthcare and give essential humanness to your existing knowledge and skills. Like all other humans, healthcare professionals are actually quite extraordinary in their ordinary humanness. This humanness is to be honoured as an empowering force for healthcare professionals and clients, and for people generally. When you reflect on honouring humanity and embodying the qualities of humanness in therapeutic relationships with the clients in your care, you accentuate opportunities for creating genuine person to person interactions, simply by practising your healthcare profession.

Author's reflection

It seems such a simple and taken for granted thing, to be human. When I reflect on my own life, I can see that I didn't really *get* this idea – what it means to be human – until the second year of my nurse training days. Even then, it was a rudimentary awakening; an insight I have been refining all of my life, I guess.

When I was in the first year of my nurse training, I was so very conscientious and absolutely driven, to be constantly doing things for people in my care. I was only 17, and frightened most of the time, of so many people and things around me. I was scared of my senior nurses, most of the doctors and very much afraid of the matron. All of these people knew more than me and had power over me. I was also afraid of so many things, such as making mistakes, failing exams, not measuring up to being a good nurse, and so on. However, I learned to not be afraid of the people in the beds, the patients. At first, they frightened me – maybe not them as people – but they were sources of fear, in remembering their diagnoses, the recall of which was tested by the senior nurses daily, and in being the ones receiving care, the ones to whom I was trying so conscientiously to 'do no harm, and do only good'. My days were spent working hard, in lifting, fetching, carrying and generally *doing* for patients, trying to be a good nurse.

I'm not too sure about the actual set of events that brought this about, but in my second year of nurse training I had the immense revelation that these *patients* in the beds were actually *people*. It seems so silly to relate now, but at that time, I was so intent on *doing for* patients, that I failed to see their personhood. The transition in my thinking came about when I returned from two days off to find that several patients for whom I had been *doing* so much, had gone home. Only a few short days before, I had been lifting them up the bed and acting generally as though they were unable to cope without me. I remember thinking then, as an 18-year-old, that I had overcompensated for these patients, and it was around about then that I slowed down inside myself, stopped running around as 'Nurse Efficiency', and took a long look at the people in the beds. I saw that they were just like me, each one was an ordinary human being propelled into extraordinary circumstances.

That was my beginning insight into looking at patients differently, and from those very early days in my career, I have been refining my awareness of what it is to be human. Years of nursing and midwifery practice later, when I was employed as an academic, I had the opportunity to undertake a PhD with my supervisor, mentor and friend, Professor Alan Pearson. He was interested in supervising research on nurse–patient relationships facilitated by what he defined as 'ordinariness', and I knew it would be a great project for me. When the project began, it was not apparent to me that this phenomenological research would uncover the qualities of being human and using humanness in providing and receiving care. It became obvious as the phenomenon emerged, but it wasn't obvious at the outset of the project. It's a bit like being human I guess. I was one – a human – so I just took it for granted. As I aged and matured emotionally and spiritually, being human meant more to me, and just as it became illuminated to some extent in my PhD, it continues to become illuminated in my personal life.

Being human for me now has a lot to do with living authentically – of not living outside myself behind a veneer or a mask – but of living as 'real' as I can be in any given moment. This means that I am getting better at apologizing, at admitting when I'm out of my depth, and at trying a little bit harder to communicate simply and clearly, so I am saying out loud what I am thinking inside. I love to be asked a question about myself and my motives, so I can try to answer it honestly and hear the response myself. Being human for me now is about being fallible, about accepting messiness and imperfection, and about being a work in progress, but it is also about claiming and valuing my humanity as an inherently good thing to embody. I don't always manage to be authentic – some days I am way off beam – just ask my family, as they get to witness my 'dark side' first hand – but, on the whole, I am pleased to say I am proud to embody the ordinary qualities of humanness and to report that my sense of connection with people and everything around me is growing day by day.

Maintaining reflective practice

Maintaining reflection will not be easy. People with the best intentions – including myself – throw reflective habits away when life overtakes them. Resolutions are actually about *hoping* for ideal circumstances. Life seldom runs to plan and many unforeseen obstructions and challenges can get in the way. When you resolve to maintain reflective processes, the trials of life may get in your way and your resolutions may not come to fruition. If this occurs, don't give in and 'throw the baby away with the bathwater'. Keep your resolution alive by holding on to the principle of the idea, even when the fine detail of your intentions goes into recess.

Affirming yourself as a reflective practitioner

To maintain reflection you may need to consider ways of affirming your intentions. Your resolution to maintain reflection may falter from time to time, but if you are assured of the value of reflection for your life and work, the central core of your intention will hold. Affirm your worth as a reflective practitioner by acknowledging your insights and how far you have come from whom and how you were when you began, to whom and how you are now. If reflective processes are working, you will be noticing some positive differences in the ways you think about your life and work. If this is so, revel in this recognition and affirm the value of your reflections.

Reflector

On what issues have you reflected since becoming a reflective practitioner? How has reflection helped you as a person and a professional?

Responding to the critiques

In Chapter 1 I acknowledged the critiques of reflective practice. Even though it has proved successful, critics have perceived limitations in such practice. To be assured of the worth of reflection, you may need to respond to the critics, so that your investment in maintaining reflection does not suffer.

For example, there has been criticism of how the nursing profession seized on the idea of reflection (Jarvis 1992), but many years have passed and it is still useful for clinicians. Greenwood (1993) took issue with Schön's idea of reflection that proposed that theories underpinning reflective activity are difficult to articulate, as they are embedded in activity itself. However, even though they are difficult to articulate, they are not impossible, as we have seen from many accounts of people who have been successful (e.g. Freshwater 2002a, 2002b; Johns 2002; Taylor *et al.* 2002).

Even though there may be a high degree of personal investment required by healthcare professionals for successful practice outcomes (Taylor 1997), if they are well prepared for reflection the positive outcomes will outweigh the risks. Barriers to learning must be overcome before we can reflect effectively (Platzer *et al.* 2000b), but these can be negotiated through guided experiences. There may be cultural barriers to empowerment through reflection (Johns 1999), but these can be identified through sensitive exploration.

Negative consequences may ensue when practitioners are pressured to reflect (Hulatt 1995), but this can be averted when personal reflection is not tied to assessment grades. Reflection may be seen to be a fundamentally flawed strategy (Mackintosh 1998), but only in some people's perceptions, so this does not invalidate it for the people with whom it has resonance. There are potential dangers in promoting 'private thoughts in public spheres' (Cotton 2001), so safeguards must be taken to ensure that reflection does not become a mechanism of social control or personal debasement. Reflective processes may have failed to 'address the postmodern, cultural contexts of reflection' (Pryce 2002), but we need to revisit notions of postmodernism and reconnect to reflection as a personal narrative that reveals local truths in a postmodern era. The criticism no longer holds that there is lack of research evidence to support the mandate to reflect (Burton 2000), as the projects are multiplying rapidly (e.g. see the references at the end of this book). Lack of research will always be cited by people who will never be satisfied with mountains of research – how much is enough?

Ghaye and Lillyman (2000) critically reviewed the foundations and criticisms of reflective practice to question whether reflective practitioners were really 'fashion victims', and having explored the limitations of it, concluded that reflective practice has a place in the postmodern world, because of its ability to explore micro-levels of human interaction and personal knowledge.

Useful processes such as reflection survive fashions and endure, long after the passage of time and trends.

Taylor (2003: 244) argued that 'reflective practice tends to adopt a naïve or romantic realist position and fails to acknowledge the ways in which reflective accounts construct the world of practice'. It is true that reflective accounts construct the world of practice, but this phenomenon is inevitable if we accept the idea that we co-create our realties. If we accept this conundrum of inevitable influence, we are left with the choice to engage or not engage with socially constructed realities. I vote for reflective practice, as it begins to work its way forward to increased insights and change. To stand still and remain unreflective is not an option if quality of patient care is to be more than rhetoric.

Be prepared to respond to critiques. There are so many ways of seeing that the slightest change of position can reveal new vistas, each with its own shortcomings. There is no end point – no nirvana – no one way of doing things. In this postmodern era we can celebrate difference and partialities. If reflective practice is seen as helpful, but not the panacea, we will benefit from what it has to offer us.

Reflector

Which of the above critiques of reflective practice hold some truth for you? How do you respond to these critiques, in order to maintain your reflective practice?

Creating a daily habit

To affirm your experience of reflection it will be important to maintain the everydayness of your reflective practice. It is easy to do something when it is novel. It is another thing to maintain a practice which has lost some of its initial appeal and requires a certain amount of discipline and attention for its continuation.

Just as you wash and feed your body as part of your essential daily activities, it is also possible to find enough space in your day-to-day life for reflection. This does not necessarily mean that you will write in a journal or speak into an audiotape every workday, but it may mean that you will be engaged sufficiently in work to reflect on it in some shape or form. In a practical sense, this may mean that you will use opportunities to take time out from the busyness of life to spend time in quietness.

Silence is the generative home of possibilities. Take time each day to find it, because it will not come to you unless you think it is important enough to seek it actively by doing nothing. It may seem like a contradiction to be active doing nothing, but unless you realize that silence is to be *claimed*, it will continue to elude you. Being busy can overtake life, so that your body rarely experiences immobility, silence and time for reflective thought. Consider the key activities of your day – simple things like washing, eating and socializing – and be alert to opportunities to be quiet, to go within and to 'just be' in the moment. From this place of quietness comes the potential for deep and effortless thought that springs up from a source of creativity and gives you clues and answers to puzzles that reside within you.

Reflector

When is your best time of day for reflection? In what ways do you seek silence in your life?

Seeing things freshly

Adopting a new way of seeing the events of everyday life can assist in maintaining reflective practice. This may mean that you try actively to keep a fresh perspective on ordinary aspects of life that you would otherwise have taken for granted. For example, what do you see when you open your eyes each morning? Have you ever really looked around the room, noticing its details? Have you ever looked carefully out the window and noticed the colours and moods of morning? As you step into active involvement in the day, start to be aware of all the little details of your life and the people with whom you interact. If these moments and people become a source of interest instead of familiarity, you may see them freshly, with new significance and potential for what and who they are and how they fit into the schemes and patterns of daily life.

Seeing the details of your life freshly will create a sense of constant connection and interest in your relationships to people and your environment. This will be excellent practice for the attentiveness you need as a reflective practitioner. For me, seeing things freshly is possible because I look out at the world from a fairly settled state inside myself, which allows me to focus on details and to be present. This way of seeing is gentle and quiet with wide, childlike eyes of interest. It is not busy and bustling, with the peering eyes of inquisitiveness for personal opportunity. Nurture a way of seeing from a quiet and steady state, which allows you to look around like a tourist visiting a foreign country for the first time. You may learn to see things freshly each day, discriminating between accepting and contesting, and making sense in general of more and more aspects of your life.

Reflector

Stop reading after this sentence and take one minute to look around to notice tiny details in your immediate environment. What benefits can you imagine in seeing things freshly in your practice environment?

Staying alert to practice

The need for seeing freshly in your personal life applies equally to your work life. You can affirm your status as a reflective practitioner by staying alert to your practice. Although you need to have a degree of comfort and familiarity with your work setting so you don't 'become a nervous wreck', too much familiarity can blind you to what is around you. Stay alert to notice the details that can keep you entrenched in unexamined clinical procedures, patterns of human relating and power plays. Work realities are complex and challenging, containing issues that relate to the need for ever-increasing technical knowledge, refinements of relationships and a constant critique of power within the organization in which you work. These issues present an immense challenge to stay alert to practice in order to monitor the moves and shifts in its nature and effects.

How do you stay alert at work? You cannot always predict how a shift at work may go. Sometimes it may be fast and action-packed and sometimes it may be slow and relatively uneventful. The point to consider is that the degree of busyness will not necessarily dictate your alertness. If you are busy you are most probably attentive to what you are doing and how you are doing it, but you may not necessarily be alert to the fine details of interactions and outcomes. This state of alertness comes when you make conscious attempts to tune in as you work. You have to be 'at the controls' and not cruising through the challenges on autopilot. Conversely, you may not be alert just because you have more time on a quiet shift. This may be the very time in which you go into a holding pattern and fail to see the fine aspects of your work, because it is 'uneventful'. The quiet shifts may be your richest times for reflection, in terms of being alert to the taken-for-granted ways of thinking, doing and being. In summary, every moment of practice is a potential source of reflection, so stay alert to these opportunities.

Reflector

Think of one example of an unexamined clinical procedure, a taken-for-granted pattern of human relating and an unchallenged work-based power play. Why have these clinical phenomena become relatively invisible and strongly entrenched in your workplace?

Finding support systems

Try to ascertain whether there are other clinicians engaged in reflective practice. You may find that there are 'closet' reflective practitioners inside your ward or unit, hospital or health region. People begin reflection through many sources, such as tertiary study, professional development courses, organizational seminars and so on. To find these people, you may need to leave a message pinned on a staff notice board, indicating that you are trying to begin a support group for reflective practitioners. You could suggest a meeting time, place and agenda and leave your contact details for the RSVP. You may be surprised who emerges out of the system.

Alternatively, you could send out an invitation on email within your organization, or on the internet, to access people more broadly and set up electronic connections with other reflective practitioners. Check the listings already in use and you may find that you could join an established group across healthcare professions and other disciplines such as education. This may lead on to organizing professional development seminars in your work setting in which to share your experiences, or getting involved in research.

Reflector

When you locate other reflective practitioners in your workplace, how will you set up regular contact and discussion?

Sharing reflection

Why not share reflective experiences in your clinic, ward, department or organization, by organizing a professional development seminar or conference? There are many possibilities. You could focus on healthcare professionals, locally, nationally or internationally. Start locally and within manageable proportions in your unit or hospital. If you decide to organize a seminar, here is a checklist of details to consider as you plan for the event:

- Venue: is it suitable and available?
- Programme: who will speak/present, for how long?
- Catering: will you provide meals and refreshments?
- Papers: will you provide participants with copies?
- Promotion: how will you invite attendance?
- Sponsorship: will you need to seek financial assistance?
- Equipment: will speakers need audio-visual aids?
- Administration: do you need a mechanism to budget and monitor numbers and costs?

Reflector

What avenues for sharing reflection are open to you? Use the checklist above to plan a seminar in your ward/unit at which you present your experiences of reflective practice.

Getting involved in research

Reflective processes work well in research projects (see Chapter 8) because the thinking required for research is similar to that required for maintaining reflective practice. Knowledge, research, thinking and reflection are related through the ways they engage people in cognitive processes.

There is wide scope for research incorporating reflective processes or centred on experiences of reflective practice. For example, you could use reflective processes as a method for data collection in the field notes of a journal, or you could construct a research proposal focused on the nature and effects of reflective practice in any work context. You could undertake research in your work setting at any level, such as a ward, department or organization. The project could involve a range of health workers. It could be planned to have a local, national or international focus and participation, depending on your knowledge and skills in establishing and maintaining research.

Reflector

Imagine a research project involving reflection. Use the formats in Chapter 8 to assist you in writing a research proposal.

Embodying reflective practice

As time passes, reflective practice will become a part of your life, so that it is in your daily repertoire. Just as you attend to the daily routines of life, so you will embody reflective practice, so that it becomes part of who and how you are. This may not mean that you remember to write in your journal or speak into an audiotape as a matter of daily routine, but it does mean that you do not lose your motivation to think reflectively and to be aware of the potential of making sense out of everyday events. You will remain aware of how life is constructed at home and work and why it might be so, and how it might be otherwise.

Your biggest challenge will be to remain aware of the danger of familiarity and the tendency to accept a given reality as though it is as it should be and could be no other way. Life will be seen as 'work in progress' in which nothing is perfect or complete and everything can be seen afresh constantly, to reveal new insights and possibilities for interpretation and adaptation. Your personal growth as a person and health professional will continue as you open yourself up to the value of your own reflections and those gained in collaboration with your colleagues. This is not to imply that life will be 'upwards and onwards' without a hitch, but you will be actively and consciously aware of the events which used to pass you by, and you will have some processes whereby you can make sense of them.

Reflector

What practical measures can you put in place to ensure that you remain aware of the danger of familiarity and the tendency to accept a given reality as though it is as it should be and could be no other way?

Summary

In this chapter I encouraged you to honour humanity in your work and I suggested that the shared affinity of being human with your clients can be therapeutic. I also suggested that if you have found reflective processes useful for your work and life, you might like to consider letting other people know about them. To this end, I discussed the value of maintaining your reflective practice by affirming yourself as a reflective practitioner, responding to the critiques, creating a daily habit, seeing things freshly, staying alert to practice, finding support systems, sharing reflection, getting involved in research and embodying reflective practice.

Final author's reflection

I have enjoyed writing this book and including these author's reflections. They have given me a chance to share something of myself with you, so that I am not just a name on the cover of your book. My reflections don't tell you every-thing about me, of course, because writing allows me to filter messages and to discriminate the level of self-disclosure I am happy to reveal to you.

I am really enjoying my retirement, which comes to me as a reward for 40 years of full-time work in nursing and health. I am finding the time and space to just *be*, to live a less structured life, with a lot less responsibility for other people, and to enjoy simple things, like coexisting gently with my part-ner, son, our two cats and geriatric dog. Metaphors of nurturance and growth are coming to life, as I tend daily to our garden and nurture my soul in lots of deep sleep and meditation. Yes, life is good. I deserve this time and space to live and reflect and I accept it gladly. I am also grateful to the publishers of this book for encouraging me to write this edition. It has been good for me to review the second edition and broaden it to include all healthcare profes-sionals. I wish you a happy and contented life, full of the rewards of reflection.

References

Anderson, J.M. (ed.) (1996) *Thinking Management: Contemporary Approaches for Nurse Managers*. Melbourne: Ausmed Publications.

Anderson, M. and Branch, M. (2000) Storytelling: a tool to promote critical reflection in the RN student, *Minority Nurse Newsletter*, 71: 1–2.

Argyris, C. and Schön, D.A. (1974) *Theory in Practice: Increasing Professional Effectiveness*. Washington, DC: Jossey-Bass.

Argyris, C., Putnam, R. and Smith, D.M. (1985) Quoted in H.S. Kim (1999) Critical reflective inquiry for knowledge development in nursing practice, *Journal of Advanced Nursing*, 29(5): 1205–12.

Azapagic, A., Perdan, S. and Clift, R. (2004) *Sustainable Development in Practice: Case Studies for Engineers and Scientists*. New York: Wiley.

Bandman, E.L. and Bandman, B. (1995) *Critical Thinking in Nursing*, 2nd edn. Norwalk, CT: Appleton & Lange.

Barrett, P. (2001) The early mothering project: what happened when the words 'action research' came to life for a group of midwives, in P. Reason and H. Bradbury (eds) *Handbook of Action Research*. London: Sage.

Baudrillard, J. (ed.) (1988) *Selected Writings Poster*. Stanford, CA: Stanford University Press.

Beirne, M. (2006) *Empowerment and Innovation: Managers, Principles and Reflective Practice*. Cheltenham: Edward Elgar Publishing.

Benner, P. and Wrubel, J. (1989) *The Primacy of Caring: Stress and Coping in Health and Illness*. Menlo Park, CA: Addison-Wesley.

Beres, L. (2002) *Romance, Suffering and Hope: Reflective Practice with Abused Women*. Toronto: University of Toronto Publishers.

Bolton, G. (2005) *Reflective Practice: Writing and Professional Development*. Thousand Oaks, CA: Sage.

Boud, D., Keogh, R. and Walker, D. (1985) *Reflection: Turning Experience into Learning*. London: Kogan Page.

Boyd, E.M. and Fales, A.W. (1983) Reflective learning key to learning from experience, *Journal of Humanistic Psychology*, 23(2): 99–117.

Bradley, A. (2006) *Personal Development and Reflective Practice in a Learning Disability Service*. London: British Institute of Learning Disabilities.

Brody, J.K. (1988) Virtue ethics caring and nursing, *Scholarly Inquiry for Nursing Practice: An International Journal*, 2(2): 87–101.

Brown, J. (2006) *A Leader's Guide to Reflective Practice*. Victoria, BC: Trafford Publishing.

Burgoyne, J. and Reynolds, M. (1997) *Management Learning: Integrating Perspectives in Theory and Practice*. Thousand Oaks, CA: Sage.

Burton, A. (2000) Reflection: nursing's practice and education panacea? *Journal of Advanced Nursing*, 31(5): 1009–17.

Card, C. (1990) Caring and evil, *Hypatia*, 5(1): 101–8.

Carr, W. and Kemmis, S. (1984) *Becoming Critical: Knowing through Action Research*. Victoria: Deakin University Press.

Carroll, J.W. (1986) *Ministry As Reflective Practice: A New Look at the Professional Model*. Herndon, VA: Alban Institute Publishers.

Carroll, J.W. and Carroll, J.S. (1991) *As One with Authority: Reflective Leadership in Ministry*. Portland, OR: Westminster John Knox Press.

Cartwright, T. (2007) *Developing Your Intuition: A Guide to Reflective Practice*. New York: Center for Creative Leadership.

Chadwick, C. and Tovey, P. (2001) *Developing Reflective Practice for Preachers*. Cambridge: Grove Books.

Chaharbaghi, K. (2004) *The Discipline, Study and Practice of Management: A Reflective Inquiry*. Bingley: Emerald Group Publishers.

Chein, I., Cook, S. and Harding, J. (1948) The field of action research, *American Psychology*, 3: 43–50.

Chenoweth, L. and Kilstoff, K. (1998) Facilitating positive changes in community dementia management through participatory action research, *International Journal of Nursing Practice*, 4: 175–88.

Cherry, N.L. (2008) *Developing Reflective Practice*. Melbourne: RMIT University Press.

Clarke, A.L. and Reading, R.P. (1994) *Endangered Species Recovery: Finding the Lessons, Improving the Process*, 2nd edn. Bermuda: Island Press.

Clegg, S. (2000) Knowing through reflective practice in higher education, *Education Action Research*, 8(3): 451–69.

Cook, D.J. (1998) Caring for the critically ill patient: past present and future, *The Journal of the American Medical Association*, 280(2): 181–2.

Cooper, A., Hetherington, R. and Katz, I. (2003) *The Risk Factor: Making the Child Protection System Work for Children*. New York: Demos Publishers.

Corey, G. (2008) *Theory and Practice of Counseling and Psychotherapy*. Florence, KY: Thompson Brooks/Cole.

Cotton, A. (2001) Private thoughts in public spheres: issues in reflection and reflective practices in nursing, *Journal of Advanced Nursing*, 36(4): 512–19.

Couch, R.F. (2004) *Reflective Practice in Occupational Therapy: A Case Study of the*

Experience at the University of Liverpool. Liverpool: University of Liverpool Publishers.

Cruickshank, D. (1996) The 'art' of reflection: using drawing to uncover knowledge development in student nurses, *Nurse Education Today*, 16(2): 127–30.

Curzer, H.J. (1993) Is care a virtue for health care professionals? *Journal of Medicine and Philosophy*, 18: 51–69.

Dallos, R. and Stedmon, J. (2009) *Reflective Practice in Psychotherapy and Counselling*. Maidenhead: McGraw-Hill Education.

Daniels, N. (1996) *Justice and Justification: Reflective Equilibrium in Theory and Practice*. Cambridge: Cambridge University Press.

Davies, M. (2002) *The Blackwell Companion to Social Work*. New York: Wiley-Blackwell.

Day, L., Pringle P. and Healy, K. (2001) *Reflective Enquiry into Therapeutic Institutions*. London: Karnac Books.

Deery, R. and Kirkham, M. (2000) Moving from hierarchy to collaboration: the birth of an action research project, *Practising Midwife*, 3(8): 25–8.

Dick, R.A. (1995) A beginner's guide to action research, *ARCS Newsletter*, 1(1): 5–9.

Dimendberg, E. and Lerup, L. (2002) *Excluded Middle: Toward a Reflective Architecture and Urbanism*. Paris: Rice School of Architecture.

Dolan, P., Canavan, J. and Pinkerton, J. (2006) *Family Support as Reflective Practice*. London: Jessica Kingsley.

Doyle, D., Hanks, G., Cherny, N.I. and Calman, K. (2005) *Oxford Textbook of Palliative Medicine*. Oxford: Oxford University Press.

Dreyfus, H.I. (1979) *What Computers Can't Do: The Limits of Artificial Intelligence*. New York: Harper & Row.

Drinka, T.J.K. and Clark, P.G. (2000) *Health Care Teamwork: Interdisciplinary Practice and Teaching*. Santa Barbara, CA: Greenwood Publishing Group.

Duffy, E. (1995) Horizontal violence: a conundrum for nursing, *Collegian*, 2(2): 5–17.

Duindam, V. and Spruijt, E. (1997) Caring fathers in the Netherlands, *Sex Roles: A Journal of Research*, 36(3–4): 14–22.

Dyck, D.L. (1997) *Teaching Engineering Writing: Using Reflective Practice to Shape Engineering Writing Pedagogy*. Columbia, SC: University of South Carolina Press.

Ehrenreich, B. and English, D. (1973) *Witches, Midwives and Nurses: A History of Women Healers*. London: Writers and Readers Publishing Cooperative.

Ekman, P. (2004) *Emotions Revealed: Recognizing Faces and Feelings to Improve Communication and Emotional Life*. New York: Henry Holt & Co.

Fay, B. (1987) *Critical Social Science: Liberation and its Limits*. Cambridge: Polity Press.

Fitzgerald, C.G. (1993) *The Supervision of Congregational Ministries: The Reflective Practice of Ministry*. Decatur, GA: Pastoral Care Publications.

Fraser, D.M. (2000) Action research to improve the pre-registration midwifery curriculum Part 1: an appropriate methodology, *Midwifery*, 16(3): 213–23.

Freidson, E. (1970) *Profession of Medicine A Study of the Sociology of Applied Knowledge.* New York: Harper & Row.

Freshwater, D. (1999a) Clinical supervision, reflective practice and guided discovery: clinical supervision, *British Journal of Nursing*, 8(20): 1383–9.

Freshwater, D. (1999b) Communicating with self through caring: the student nurse's experience of reflective practice, *International Journal of Human Caring*, 3(3): 28–33.

Freshwater, D. (2001) Critical reflexivity: a politically and ethically engaged method for nursing, *NT Research*, 6(1): 526–37.

Freshwater, D. (2002a) Guided reflection in the context of post-modern practice, in C. Johns (ed.) *Guided Reflection: Advancing Practice*. Oxford: Blackwell Science.

Freshwater, D. (ed.) (2002b) *Therapeutic Nursing: Improving Patient Care through Reflection*. London: Sage.

Freshwater, D., Taylor, B. and Sherwood, D. (2008) *International Textbook of Reflective Practice in Nursing*. Oxford: Blackwell.

Fry, S. (1989) Toward a theory of nursing ethics, *Advances in Nursing Science*, 11(4): 9–22.

Gardner, I. and Boucher, C. (2000) *Reflective Practice as a Meta-competency for Australian Allied Health Managers*. Melbourne: RMIT Business Press.

Gelpi, D.L. (1998) *The Conversion Experience: A Reflective Process for RCIA Participants and Others*. Mahwah, NJ: Paulist Press.

Ghaye, T. (2005) *Developing the Reflective Healthcare Team*. Oxford: Wiley-Blackwell.

Ghaye, T. and Lillyman, S. (2000) Reflections on Schön: fashion victims or joining up practice with theory? in *Reflection: Principles and Practice for Healthcare Professionals*. London: Quay Books.

Ghaye, T. and Lillyman, S. (2006) *Learning Journals and Critical Incidents: Reflective Practice for Health Care Professionals*. London: Quay Books.

Gilbert, T. (2001) Reflective practice and supervision: meticulous rituals of the confessional, *Journal of Advanced Nursing*, 36(2): 199–205.

Gilligan, C. (1977) In a different voice: women's of self and morality *Harvard Educational Review*, 47(4): 481–517.

Gilligan, C. (1982) *In a Different Voice: Psychological Theory and Women's Development*. Cambridge, MA: Harvard University Press.

Giroux, H.A. (1990) *Curriculum Discourse as Postmodernist Critical Practice*. Geelong: Deakin University Press.

Glass, N. (1997) Horizontal violence in nursing, *The Australian Journal of Holistic Nursing*, 4(1): 15–21.

Glaze, E. (2001) Reflection as a transforming process: student advanced nurse practitioners' experiences of developing reflective skills as part of an MSc programme, *Journal of Advanced Nursing*, 34: 639–47.

Golding, D. and Currie, D. (2000) *Thinking About Management: A Reflective Practice Approach*. New York: Routledge.

Goodin, R.E. (2005) *Reflective Democracy*. Oxford: Oxford University Press.

Gould, N. and Baldwin, M. (2004) *Social Work, Critical Reflection, and the Learning Organization*. Aldershot: Ashgate.

Gould, N. and Taylor, I. (1996) *Reflective Learning for Social Work: Research, Theory and Practice*. New York: Arena Publishers.

Greenwood, J. (1993) Reflective practice: a critique of the work of Argyris and Schön, *Journal of Advanced Nursing*, 18: 1183–7.

Griffin, E. (2008) *The Reflective Executive: A Spirituality of Business and Enterprise*. Eugene, OR: Wipf & Stock.

Habermas, J. (1972) *Knowledge and Human Interests*. London: Heinemann.

Handcock, P. (1999) Reflective practice: using a learning journal, *Nursing Standard*, 13(17): 37–40.

Harms, L. (2007) *Working with People: Communication Skills for Professional Practice*. Oxford: Oxford University Press.

Heath, H. and Freshwater, D. (2000) Clinical supervision as an emancipatory process: avoiding inappropriate intent, *Journal of Advanced Nursing*, 32(5): 1298–306.

Heidegger, M. (1962) *Being and Time*, trans J. Macquarrie and E. Robinson. New York: Harper & Row.

Hoagland, S. (1991) Some thoughts about caring, in C. Card (ed.) *Feminist Ethics*. Lawrence, KS: University Press of Kansas.

Hoare, C. (2006) *Handbook of Adult Development and Learning*. New York: Oxford University Press.

Hookins, M., Pike, N. and Rhodes, P. (2009) *Developing Reflective Practice in Social Work: A Critical Approach*. Thousand Oaks, CA: Sage.

Hoshmand, L.T. (1994) *Orientation to Inquiry in a Reflective Professional Psychology*. New York: SUNY Press.

Houston, J. (1990) *The Search for the Beloved: Journeys in Sacred Psychology*. Los Angeles: J. P. Tharcher.

Hughes, B. (2001) *Evolutionary Playwork and Reflective Analytic Practice*. New York: Routledge.

Hulatt, I. (1995) A sad reflection, *Nursing Standard*, 9(20): 22–3.

Jarvis, P. (1992) Reflective practice in nursing, *Nursing Education Today*, 12: 174–81.

Jasper, M. 2003 *Beginning Reflective Practice*. Cheltenham: Nelson Thornes.

Johns, C. (1999) Reflection as empowerment? *Nursing Inquiry*, 6(4): 241–9.

Johns, C. (2000) Working with Alice: a reflection, *Complementary Therapies in Nursing and Midwifery*, 6: 199–303.

Johns, C. (ed.) (2002) *Guided Reflection: Advancing Practice*. Oxford: Blackwell Science.

Johns, C. (2003) Easing into the light, *International Journal for Human Caring*, 7(1): 49–55.

Jourard, S.M. (1971) *The Transparent Self*. New York: D. Van Nostrand.

Keatinge, D., Scarfe, C., Bellchambers, H., McGee, J., Oakham, R., Probert, C.,

Stewart, L. and Stokes, J. (2000) The manifestation and nursing management of agitation in institutionalised residents with dementia, *International Journal of Nursing Practice*, 6: 16–25.

Kemmis, S. and McTaggart, R. (eds) (1988) *The Action Research Planner*, 3rd edn. Geelong: Deakin University Press.

Kim, H.S. (1999) Critical reflective inquiry for knowledge development in nursing practice, *Journal of Advanced Nursing*, 29(5): 1205–12.

Kinsella, E.A. (2000) *Professional Development and Reflective Practice: Strategies for Learning Through Professional Experience: A Workbook for Practitioners*. Ottawa: CAOT Publications.

Kitchen, P.R.B. (2002) *Experiential Learning and Reflective Practice in Medicine and Ministry*. Melbourne: Melbourne College of Divinity Publishers.

Kitzinger, S. (1991) Why women need midwives, in S. Kitzinger (ed.) *The Midwife Challenge*. London: Pandora.

Knott, C. and Scragg, T. (2007) *Reflective Practice in Social Work*. Exeter: Learning Matters.

Koch, T., Kralik, D. and Kelly, S. (2000) We just don't talk about it: men living with urinary incontinence and multiple sclerosis, *International Journal of Nursing Practice*, 6: 253–60.

Lewin, K. (1946) Action research and minority issues, *Journal of Social Issues*, 2: 34–46.

Leyden, A.T. (2004) *Primary Care Physicians in Reflective Practice: Learning to Treat Depression*. New York: Columbia University.

MacAuley, D., Clarke, R. and Croft, P. (1998) *Critical Reading for the Reflective Practitioner: A Guide for Primary Care*. New York: Butterworth-Heinemann.

MacIntyre, A. (1984) *After Virtue*. Notre Dame: University of Notre Dame Press.

Mackintosh, C. (1998) Reflection: a flawed strategy for the nursing profession, *Nurse Education Today*, 18: 553–7.

Markham, T. (2002) Response to 'private thoughts in public spheres: issues in reflection and reflective practices in nursing', *Journal of Advanced Nursing*, 38(3): 286–7.

Martyn, H. and Atkinson, M. (2000) *Developing Reflective Practice: Making Sense of Social Work in a World of Change*. Bristol: The Policy Press.

Mayeroff, M. (1971) *On Caring*. New York: Harper & Row.

McCool, W. and McCool, S. (1989) Feminism and nurse-midwifery: historical overview and current issues, *Journal of Nurse-Midwifery*, 345(6): 323–34.

McDermott, F. (2003) *Inside Group Work: A Guide to Reflective Practice*. Melbourne: Allen & Unwin.

McKinlay, L. and Ross, H. (2008) *You and Others: Reflective Practice for Group Effectiveness in Human Services*. Toronto: Pearson Education.

McMorland, J. and Piggott-Irvine, E. (2000) Facilitation as midwifery: facilitation and praxis in group learning, *Systematic Practice and Action Research*, 13(2): 121–38.

Mezirow, J. (1981) A critical theory of adult learning and education, *Adult Education*, 32: 3–24.

Mickelson, K.M. (2002) *The Social Construction of Reflective Practice*. Madison, WI: University of Wisconsin.

Miller, S. (2007) *Keeping It Together: A Reflective Practice Tool for Faith-Based Community Development Practitioners*. London: Faith Based Regeneration Network Publishers.

Morgan, G. (2006) *Images of Organization*. Thousand Oaks, CA: Sage.

Munroe, J., Ford, H., Scott, A., Furnival, E., Andrews, S. and Grayson, S. (2002) Action research responding to midwives' views of different methods of fetal monitoring in labour, *MIDIRS Midwifery Digest*, 12(4): 495–8.

Munson, T.N. (1976) *Reflective Theology: Philosophical Orientations in Religion*. Santa Barbara, CA: Greenwood Press.

Murray, E. and Simpson, J. (2000) *Professional Development and Management for Therapists: An Introduction*. New York: Wiley-Blackwell.

Noddings, N. (1984) *A Feminine Approach to Ethics and Moral Education*. Berkeley, CA: University of California Press.

Normore, A. (2009) *Leadership for Social Justice: Promoting Equity and Excellence Through Inquiry and Reflective Practice*. Birmingham: IAP Publishers.

Oakley, A. and Houd, S. (1990) *Helpers in Childbirth: Midwifery Today*. New York: Hemisphere Publishing.

Oliver, M. (2007) *Pastoral Care, Counselling and Support: Reflective Practice in Palliative Care: A Resource Manual for Health Professionals*. Adelaide: University of South Australia.

Osofsky, J.D. and Fitzgerald, H.E. (1999) *Handbook of Infant Mental Health: Early Intervention, Evaluation, and Assessment*. New York: Wiley.

Payne, M. and Campling, J. (2005) *Modern Social Work Theory*. Chicago: Lyceum Books.

Pearson, A. (ed.) (1988) *Primary Nursing*. London: Croom Helm.

Pearson, A., Borbasi, S., Fitzgerald, M., Kowanko, I. and Walsh, K. (1997) *Evidence Based Nursing: An Examination of Nursing Within the International Evidence Based Health Care Practice Movement*. Sydney: RCNA Discussion Document no. 1, *Nursing Review*.

Pellicer, L.O. (2007) *Caring Enough to Lead: How Reflective Practice Leads to Moral Leadership*. Newbury Park, CA: Corwin Press.

Pitts, J. (2007) *Portfolios, Personal Development and Reflective Practice*. USA: ASME Publishers.

Platzer, H., Blake, D. and Ashford, D. (2000a) Barriers to learning from reflection: a study of the use of groupwork with post-registration nurses, *Journal of Advanced Nursing*, 31(5): 1001–8.

Platzer, H., Blake, D. and Ashford, D. (2000b) An evaluation of process and outcomes from learning through reflective practice groups on a post-registration nursing course, *Journal of Advanced Nursing*, 31(3): 689–95.

Polit, D., Beck, C. and Hungler, B. (2001) *Essentials of Nursing Research: Methods, Appraisal, and Utilization*. Philadelphia, PA: Lippincott.

Poulter, S.J.H. (2001) *Issues of Reflective Practice and Organisational Learning in the Protective Investigation of Child Sexual Abuse*. Melbourne: Monash University Press.

Pryce, A. (2002) Refracting experience: reflection, postmodernity and transformations, *NT Research*, 7(4): 298–311.

Puka, B. (1990) The liberation of caring: a different voice for Gilligan's 'different voice', *Hypatia*, 5(1): 55–82.

Puka, B. (1991) The science of caring, *Hypatia*, 6(2): 200–10.

Redmond, B. (2006) *Reflection in Action: Developing Reflective Practice in Health and Social Services*. Aldershot: Ashgate.

Renninger, K.A. and Sigel, I.E. (eds) (2006) *Handbook of Child Psychology: Child Psychology in Practice*. New York: Wiley.

Robb, M., Barrett S. and Komaromy, C. (2004) *Communication, Relationships and Care: A Reader*. New York: Routledge.

Rolfe, G. (2003) Is there a place for reflection in the nursing curriculum? A reply to Newell, *Clinical Effectiveness in Nursing*, 7(1): 61.

Rosenau, P. (1992) *Post-modernism and the Social Sciences: Insights, Inroads and Intrusions*. Princeton, NJ: Princeton University Press.

Ruch, G.M. (2004) *Reflective Practice in Contemporary Child Care Social Work*. Southampton: University of Southampton.

Rustin, M. and Bradley, J. (2008) *Work Discussion: Learning from Reflective Practice in Work with Children and Families*. London: Karnac Books.

Sargent, M. (2001) Move with the times – reflection is here to stay in nurse education, *Nursing Standard*, 16(13–14–15): 30.

Schön, D.A. (1983) *The Reflective Practitioner: How Practitioners Think in Action*. New York: Basic Books.

Schön, D.A. (1987) *Educating the Reflective Practitioner*. London: Jossey-Bass.

Segal, S. (2006) *The Reflective Practice of Managers and Leaders: The Cases of Steve Waugh and Andrew Grove*. Sydney: Macquarie Graduate School of Management Publishers.

Senge, P.M. (2006) *The Fifth Discipline: The Art and Practice of the Learning Organization*. New York: Doubleday/Currency.

Shapiro, K.J. (1985) *Bodily Reflective Modes: A Phenomenological Method for Psychology*. Durham, NC: Duke University Press.

Shorten, A. and Wallace, M. (1997) Evidence based practice: the future is clear, *Australian Nursing Journal*, 4(6): 22–4.

Sik, M.C. (1997) *Transition from Missionary Leadership to Leadership by a Team of Nationals: A Reflective Study of a Taiwan Experience*. Taiwan: Trinity Evangelical Divinity School Press.

Smyth, W.J. (1986a) *Reflection-in-action EED432 Educational Leadership in Schools*. Geelong: Deakin University Press.

Smyth, W.J. (1986b) The reflective practitioner in nursing education, unpublished paper presented to the Second National Nursing Education Seminar, SACAE, Adelaide.

Soares, S.M.S. (2005) *Reflective Practice in Medicine*. Rotterdam: Erasmus Universiteit.

Sternberg, R.J. and Horvath, J.A. (1999) *Tacit Knowledge in Professional Practice: Researcher and Practitioner Perspectives*. Philadelphia, PA: Lawrence Erlbaum Associates.

Stickley, T. and Freshwater, D. (2002) The art of loving and the therapeutic relationship, *Nursing Inquiry*, 9(4): 250–6.

Street, A. (1991) *From Image to Action: Reflection in Nursing Practice*. Geelong: Deakin University Press.

Street, A. (1992) *Inside Nursing: A Critical Ethnography of Clinical Nursing*. New York: SUNY.

Streubert Speziale, H. and Rinaldi Carpenter, D. (2003) *Qualitative Research in Nursing: Advancing the Humanistic Perspective*. Philadelphia, PA: Lippincott.

Stringer, E.T. (1996) *Action Research: A Handbook for Practitioners*. Thousand Oaks, CA: Sage.

Swartz, I., Gibson, K., Richter, L. and Gelman, T. (2002) *Reflective Practice: Psychodynamic Ideas in the Community*. South Africa: HSRC Press.

Taylor, B.J. (1988) What are the patients' perceptions of the usefulness of information given to them by nurses and what are the nurses' perceptions of their roles and constraints as teachers in giving effective patient education in a postnatal ward? Research paper submitted in partial fulfilment of the requirements for the degree of Master of Education, Deakin University

Taylor, B.J. (1991) The phenomenon of ordinariness in nursing, unpublished PhD (nursing) thesis, Deakin University.

Taylor, B.J. (1997) Big battles for small gains: a cautionary note for teaching reflective processes in nursing and midwifery, *Nursing Inquiry*, 4: 19–26.

Taylor, B.J. (2000) *Reflective Practice: A Guide for Nurses and Midwives*. Buckingham: Open University Press.

Taylor, B.J. (2001) Identifying and transforming dysfunctional nurse-nurse relationships through reflective practice and action research, *International Journal of Nursing Practice*, 7(6): 406–13.

Taylor, B.J. (2002a) Technical reflection for improving nursing and midwifery procedures using critical thinking in evidence based practice, *Contemporary Nurse*, 13(2–3): 281–7.

Taylor, B.J. (2002b) Becoming a reflective nurse or midwife: using complementary therapies while practising holistically, *Complementary Therapies in Nursing and Midwifery*, 8(4): 62–8.

Taylor, B.J. (2006) *Reflective Practice: A Guide for Nurses and Midwives*, 2nd edn. Maidenhead: Open University Press.

Taylor, B.J., Bulmer, B., Hill, L., Luxford, C., McFarlane, J. and Stirling, K. (2002) Exploring idealism in palliative nursing care through reflective practice and action research, *International Journal of Palliative Nursing*, 8(7): 324–30.

Taylor, B.J., Kermode, S. and Roberts K. (2006) Research, in *Nursing and Health Care: Evidence for Practice*, 3rd edn. Sydney: Thomson Australia.

Taylor, C. (2003) Issues and innovations in nursing education – narrating practice: reflective accounts and the textual construction of reality, *Journal of Advanced Nursing*, 42(3): 244.

Thomashow, M. (1996) *Ecological Identity: Becoming a Reflective Environmentalist*. Cambridge, MA: MIT Press.

Thorpe, K. and Barsky, J. (2001) Healing through self-reflection, *Journal of Advanced Nursing*, 35(5): 760–8.

Todd, G. and Freshwater, D. (1999) Reflective practice and guided discovery: clinical supervision, *British Journal of Nursing*, 8(20): 1383–9.

United Nations Centre for Human Settlements (2005) *Key Competencies for Improving Local Governance*. Budapest: UN-HABITAT.

van Hooft, S., Gillam, L. and Byrnes, M. (1995) *Facts and Values: An Introduction to Critical Thinking for Nurses*. Sydney: Maclennan & Petty.

Warren-Adamson, C. and Ruch, G. (2008) *Post-Qualifying Child Care Social Work: Developing Reflective Practice*. Thousand Oaks, CA: Sage.

Webb, S.S. (2006) *Using Healthcare Outcome Data and Reflective Practice to Inform Microsystems of Interprofessional Practice Performance*. Knoxville, TN: University of Tennessee Health Science Center.

Wessels, T. (2006) *The Myth of Progress: Toward a Sustainable Future*. Vermont: UPNE Publishers.

Wilkinson, J.M. (1996) *Nursing Process: A Critical Thinking Approach*. Menlo Park, CA: Addison-Wesley Nursing.

Wilson, J. (2005) *Human Resource Development: Learning & Training for Individuals & Organizations*. London: Kogan Page.

Yelloly, M. and Henkel, M. (1995) *Learning and Teaching in Social Work: Towards Reflective Practice*. London: Jessica Kingsley.

Young, A.P. and Cooke, M. (2002) *Managing and Implementing Decisions in Health Care: Six Steps to Effective Management Series*. Oxford: Elsevier Health Sciences.

Yu, S.W.K. and Chau, R.C.M. (1997) The sexual division of labour in mainland China and Hong Kong, *International Journal of Urban and Regional Research*, 21(4): 607–20.

Zammit, C. (2008) The lived experience of dying: a reflective topical auto-biography, PhD thesis awarded posthumously, Southern Cross University, Australia.

Index